Copyright 2020 by Arnetta Ware -All rights reserved.

No part of this publication may be reproduced, distributed, or transmitted in any form or by any means, including photocopying, recording, or other electronic or mechanical methods, without the prior written permission of the publisher, except in the case of brief quotations embodied in reviews and certain other non-commercial uses permitted by copyright law.

This Book is provided with the sole purpose of providing relevant information on a specific topic for which every reasonable effort has been made to ensure that it is both accurate and reasonable. Nevertheless, by purchasing this Book you consent to the fact that the author, as well as the publisher, are in no way experts on the topics contained herein, regardless of any claims as such that may be made within. It is recommended that you always consult a professional prior to undertaking any of the advice or techniques discussed within. This is a legally binding declaration that is considered both valid and fair by both the Committee of Publishers Association and the American Bar Association and should be considered as legally binding within the United States.

CONTENTS

- INTRODUCTION 5
- THE KETOGENIC DIET 6
- PIZZA RECIPES 9
  - 1. Chewy Low-Carb Pizza Crust 9
  - 2. Crunchy Cheese Pizza 10
  - 3. Flatbread Keto Pizza Recipe 11
  - 4. Cheese Crust Pizza 12
  - 5. Alternate Crust Pepperoni Pizza 13
  - 6. Vegetarian Pizza 14
  - 7. Sausage Crust Pizza 15
  - 8. Thin Crust White Pizza 16
  - 9. StLouis-Style Pizza 17
  - 10. New-York style pizza 18
  - 11. New Haven-Style Clam Pizza 19
  - 12. Greece-style Pizza 20
  - 13. Vegan Bacon Fat Head Pizza 21
  - 14. Mushroom-Basil Pizza 22
  - 15. BBQ Tempeh Pizza 23
  - 16. Tofu & Vegan Bacon Ranch Pizza 24
  - 17. Kale-Artichoke Pizza 25
  - 18. Tomato-Vegan Bacon Pizza 26
  - 19. Mushroom-Pepper Pizza 27
  - 20. Vegetarian Spinach-Olive Pizza 28
  - 21. Cauliflower-Vegan Bacon Pizza Casserole 29
  - 22. Italian Mushroom Pizza 30
  - 23. Extra Cheesy Pizza 31
  - 24. Spicy and Smoky Pizza 32
  - 25. Taco pizza 33
  - 26. Broccoli-Pepper Pizza 34
  - 27. Caramelized Onion and Ricotta cheese Pizza 35
  - 28. Tofu Scampi Pizza 36
  - 29. Strawberry-Tomato Pizza 37
  - 30. Mediterranean Pizza 38
  - 31. Pesto Arugula Pizza 39
  - 32. Four Cheese Mexican Pizza 40
  - 33. Chicago style thin-crust Pizza 41
  - 34. Regina Pizza 42
  - 35. Margherita Pizza 43
  - 36. Marinara Pizza 44
  - 37. Napoli Pizza with Anchovies 45
  - 38. Capricciosa Pizza 46
  - 39. Pizza Frittata 47
  - 40. Keto Gluten-Free Pizza Crust 48

41. Personal Pan Pizza Crusts 49
42. Egg and Gluten-Free Pizza 50
43. Pizza Ball Head 51
44. Keto Pizza with Chicken and Garlic 52
45. High-protein Pizza Cabbage with Nutri-plus 53
46. Pulled Pork with Pineapple 54

PASTA RECIPES 55
47. Creamy Zoodles 55
48. Keto Ricotta Gnocchi 56
49. Keto Carbonara Pasta 57
50. Fresh Egg Pasta 58
51. Palmini Low-Carb Pasta 59
52. Keto Shirataki Noodles 60
53. Keto Butter Cabbage Noodles 61
54. Keto Shrimp Scampi 62
55. Vietnamese Pasta Bowl 63
56. Keto Japanese Seafood Pasta 64
57. Low carb Spaghetti & Fettuccine 65
58. Low carb fettuccine Alfredo (with Brussel sprouts or roasted broccoli) 66
59. Low carb Lasagna (with cucumber salad or sautéed spinach) 67
60. Keto lasagna (with roasted cauliflower or roasted broccoli). 68
61. Fathead low carb gnocchi (with basil pesto or mushroom cream sauce).... 69
62. Fathead low carb gnocchi (with basil pesto or mushroom cream sauce).... 70
63. Low carb egg pasta 71
64. Low carb pasta 72
65. Low carb pasta (with basil pesto); 73
66. Cheese head lasagna sheets 74
67. Faux egg noodles 75
68. Stove made Keto Cauliflower Mac and cheese 76
69. Kelp noodle salad 77
70. Kelp noodles (with sesame chicken). 78
71. Palmini noodles (with sausage ragu). 79
72. Butternut squash noodles. 80
73. Shirataki noodles (with mushrooms) 81
74. Creamy Zoodles 82
75. Butternut squash noodles (with mushroom cream sauce) 83
76. Shirataki noodles (with coconut Basil chicken) 84
77. Rosemary lasagna noodles 85
78. Baked Zucchini Noodles with Feta 86
79. Cauli Mac-n-Cheese 87
80. Crispy Bacon and Sage Carbonara Zoodles 88
81. Edamame Kelp Noodles 89
82. Chinese Seitan and Celeriac Noodles 90
83. Garlic Pecorino Koodles with Tofu 91
84. Creamy Tuscan Tofu Linguine 92

85. One-Pot Spicy Cheddar Pasta 93
86. Mushroom Alfredo Zoodles 94
87. Tomato Kale Eggplant Skillet with Keto Linguine 95
88. Mustard Tofu Shirataki 96
89. Lemon Chicken with Angel Hair Pasta 97
90. Lemon Garlic Shrimp with Zucchini Pasta 98
91. Mushroom Pasta with Shirataki Noodles 99
92. Pesto Shirataki Noodles–Vegan 100
93. Salmon Pasta 101
94. Salmon and Avocado Pesto Zucchini Noodles 102
95. Stuffed Shells Florentine 103
96. Stuffed Shells with Arrabbiata Sauce 104
97. Sunday Shrimp Pasta Bake 105
98. Creamy Zoodles 106
99. Swiss Cheese Lasagna 107
100. Swiss Macaroni 108
101. Tangy Meatballs Over Noodles 109
102. Tasty Chicken Noodle Casserole 110
103. Tempting Turkey Casserole 111

INTRODUCTION

Okay, so we know that a ketogenic diet is characterized by low-carb, medium-protein, and high-fat intake. The combination of these three ingredients will cause the body to go into ketosis. Ketosis is a metabolic shift in the body in a way that allows the body to burn fat rather than carbohydrates.

The carbohydrates that are consumed are converted into glucose and insulin. Here, glucose is basically sugar. Glucose is the most convenient source of energy because your body can convert it to energy easier. As such, the body prefers using that up first. Another byproduct of carbohydrates is insulin, which is a hormone produced by your pancreas. This hormone helps process glucose in your body by transporting the glucose in the body to where it is needed. When your body has enough energy, the excess glucose will be converted to adipose tissue, or fat, as a backup. Of course, that does not mean that the body uses that fat first if there are carbohydrates available.

You see, the fat in your body is considered to be the backup source of power. Therefore, in a normal situation, your body would burn carbohydrates, then fats, then proteins, in that order. As such, the body does not burn fat as effectively. Ketosis promotes weight loss by making the body prioritize burning fat, thus resulting in more fat being burned.

Many ordinary diets contain plenty of carbohydrates, which are not bad in itself. It is only bad when you take in more energy than you spend it, which means you create an energy leftover which would be converted to fat. Day by day, your weight adds up very quickly. For such a diet, glucose is the main source of energy because it contains plenty of it. However, the glucose in your body can only last you a few days. Your body will convert glucose to fat if you do not use glucose up. So, when your glucose store runs dry in a few days, your body will switch to another source of energy through a biochemical process known as ketogenesis.

When this process starts, your liver starts to take the fat in your body and break it down, creating an alternative source of energy. When that happens, your ketone level goes up and your body. This is the moment when you enter ketosis.

How to Enter Ketosis

You have a few options when it comes to entering ketosis.

The most direct one is by depriving your body of carbohydrates, therefore glucose, through fasting for a long period of time. When you stop eating altogether, your body will turn to burn fat as a source of energy because it has no glucose to work with. But of course, fasting and intermittent fasting is a whole different subject on its own and we will not cover that in this book. But do remember that fasting has its caveat.

Another option is to eat less. You just have to consume less than 20 to 50 grams of your daily carbohydrate intake a day. This will depend on who is fasting. Some require fewer while some require more, perhaps even more than 50 grams. However, the bottom line is that people who are on a keto diet only consume 5% of their usual carbohydrate intake.

But whatever method you use, it all boils down to this:

Cut down on carbs intake to 5% of regular intake

Increase fat intake to 80%

The lack of carbs will force the body to burn fat instead

When the ketone level in your blood rises high enough, you enter a state of ketosis

Profit.

THE KETOGENIC DIET

The ketogenic diet is a standard dietary treatment that was created to recreate the achievement and expel the constraints of the non-standard utilization of fasting to treat epilepsy. Albeit famous during the 1920s and '30s, it was generally surrendered for new anticonvulsant drugs. Most people with epilepsy can effectively control their seizures with medication. Nonetheless, 20–30% neglect to accomplish such control in spite of attempting various medications.

The ketogenic diet is a high-fat, sufficient protein, low-sugar diet that in medication is utilized fundamentally to get troublesome control (recalcitrant) epilepsy in kids. The diet powers the body to consume fats as opposed to starches. Typically, the sugars contained in food are changed over into glucose, which is then shipped around the body and is especially significant in powering mind work. In any case, if little sugar stays in the diet, the liver proselyte's fat into unsaturated fats and ketone bodies. The ketone bodies go into the cerebrum and supplant glucose as a vitality source. A raised degree of ketone bodies in the blood, a state known as ketosis, prompts a decrease in the recurrence of epileptic seizures. Around half of kids and youngsters with epilepsy who have attempted some type of this diet saw the quantity of seizures drop by in any event half, and the impact continues significantly subsequent to ceasing the diet.[2] Some proof demonstrates that grown-ups with epilepsy may profit by the diet, and that a less exacting routine, for example, an adjusted Atkins diet, is also viable. Potential reactions may incorporate obstruction, elevated cholesterol, development easing back, acidosis, and kidney stones.

The first helpful diet for pediatric epilepsy gives simply enough protein to body development and fix, and adequate calories to keep up the right weight for age and stature. The great remedial ketogenic diet was created for the treatment of pediatric epilepsy during the 1920s and was generally utilized in the following decade, yet its prominence melted away with the presentation of compelling anticonvulsant meds. This great ketogenic diet contains a 4:1 proportion by weight of fat to consolidated protein and starch. This is accomplished by barring high-carb foods, for example, boring products of the soil, bread, pasta, grains, and sugar while expanding the utilization of foods high in fat, for example, nuts, cream, and margarine. Most dietary fat is made of atoms called long-chain triglycerides (LCTs). In any case, medium-chain triglycerides (MCTs)— produced using unsaturated fats with shorter carbon chains than LCTs—are more ketogenic. A variation of the great diet known as the MCT ketogenic diet utilizes a type of coconut oil, which is rich in MCTs, to give around a large portion of the calories. As less by and large fat is required in this variation of the diet, a more prominent extent of starches and protein can be devoured, permitting a more noteworthy assortment of food decisions.

Conceivable restorative uses for the ketogenic diet have been read for some extra neurological issue, some of which include: Alzheimer's ailment, amyotrophic sidelong sclerosis, migraine, neurotrauma, torment, Parkinson's illness, and rest issue.

Another main explanation individual go keto is supported vitality. At the point when you don't eat plentiful measures of carbs, levels of insulin—the hormone that controls glucose—stay a lot steadier than they do on the starch-based diet a great many people are utilized to. At the point when your glucose is steady, you don't have evening vitality crashes that make you need to nod off at your work area. An examination in the Annals of Internal Medicine indicated that a ketogenic diet-controlled glucose more successfully than a progressively standard, low-calorie diet that was high in carbs.

Keto diets may likewise cause it simpler to consume additional fat off your waistline. Research from 2013 in the British Journal of Nutrition found that keto dieters lost more weight long haul than the individuals who ate a low-fat diet.

The positives of the Ketogenic Diet

Blood Sugar Control

Starchy foods and sugary foods produce sugars in the body. This is why people with diabetes suffer, and to my surprise, in the past, meal plans created for people with diabetes were loaded with carbohydrates, fruits, and processed milk. So wrong!

By avoiding carbohydrates, the amount of sugars in the body drops drastically, which requires a relative reduction in the use of diabetic medication.

Significant enough, there are many testimonies of the Keto diet healing diabetics completely; that's some good news right there!

Weight loss

It goes without stressing that you're up for a significant weight shed once you start dieting the Keto way. Why so? Because your body now burns all the stored up fat in your body for energy.

Like I said earlier when on carbs, the body's duty to consume fats gets dormant and will rather burn carbs. But, when carbohydrates are reduced, the body is moved into a metabolic state called ketosis where it is forced to burn fats.

Appetite Control

Ever wondered why there is a word as "sweet-tooth"? The more sugars you eat, the more of it you will want. Therefore, the unexpected hunger pangs after taking sugary foods or fruits.

Appetite levels increase, not necessarily, because the body needs food. It is because the body burns sugars fast and creates a false alert that it needs more food. The truth is it just needs some SUGAR.

On the keto diet, fat burns slower keeping the body fuller for an extended period. I usually find myself eating twice a day on a healthy meal because my breakfast is fat-rich and keeps me full past my lunch period sometimes. If hungry in between meals, I snack on a Keto option, and I'm good.

Energy Levels

Starch and sugars are tricky – they satisfy fast, but burn out fast. When this happens, the body is left weak and craves more carbs only to be burned quickly again. Energy levels then fluctuate causing most parts of the body to be less vibrant.

On the other hand, feeding on high fats and Proteins create a steady level of energy because fats and Protein burn gradually and in a consistent manner.

Keto Diet and Insulin Resistance

On a high carb diet, the body breaks starch into useful sugar components known as glucose, which is transported to the muscles and tissues as energy. The carrier of this glucose is insulin – meant to be a good thing.

However, in cases where the body becomes resistant to insulin, sugar breaks lose in the body. Once, the liver, cells in the muscles, and fats stop absorbing the sugars, they find their way into the blood and have a free flow – diabetes sets in.

Through the Keto diet, this problem is prevented because the body is naturally reduced of sugars through carb reduction hence there is more control over the amount of sugar needed in the body.

Why Fat and Proteins – does this mean carbohydrate are bad?

No, don't get it twisted. Carbohydrates aren't bad for the sense that they are nature's gift for feeding. However, for their starchy and sugary components, a small measure of carb intake should be considered to avoid increased sugar levels and low energy.

Fats and proteins, on the other hand, are safer options to consume in larger quantities. They are a more sustainable way of providing energy to the body, lead to weight loss, and are entirely healthy to the body.

Meanwhile, fats can be categorized into two parts: good and bad fats. Below I give examples of some good fats, but mostly these are sourced from natural ingredients like meat, fatty fish, nuts, avocados, tofu, and seeds. While bad fats are often processed products, for example, some "vegetable oils."

Concisely, you want to ensure that you are deriving your fats from natural sources and using vegetables with low carb counts if you need to eat carbohydrates like rice.

PIZZA RECIPES

1. Chewy Low-Carb Pizza Crust

Preparation time: 10 minutes Cooking time: 10 minutesServings: 6

INGREDIENTS:
- Shredded mozzarella cheese (1.5 cups)
- Salt (1 pinch)
- Grated parmesan cheese (2 tablespoons)
- Hemp seeds (.75 cup)
- Garlic powder (.5 teaspoon)
- Baking powder (.5 teaspoon)
- Eggs (3)

DIRECTIONS:
2. Warm the oven before it is time to bake to reach 350º Fahrenheit.
3. Add a layer of parchment baking paper onto a large baking sheet.
4. Combine all of the fixings in a large bowl, mixing well. Wait for about 5 minutes.
5. Using a ¼ cup measure, make six mounds of the cheese mixture on the baking sheet. Pat down it to about a .25-inch thickness.
6. Bake for 20 minutes. Cool before removing from the pans.

NUTRITION: Calories: 268 Total Fat: 20g Carbs: 2g Protein: 18g

2. .Crunchy Cheese Pizza

Preparation time: 10 minutes Cooking time: 15 minutesServings: 6

INGREDIENTS:
- Pepperoni (2 ounces)
- Mushrooms (3)
- Oregano (2 pinches - dried)
- Keto-friendly marinara sauce (2 tablespoons)
- Shredded cheddar cheese (.5 cup)
- Shredded mozzarella cheese (2 cups)
- High-heat non-stick skillet

DIRECTIONS:
1. Thinly slice the pepperoni and mushrooms. Toss onto a lined cookie sheet. Broil/grill for 3 to 5 minutes.
2. Place the pizza pan on the grill using the high-heat temperature setting. Spread the mozzarella cheese evenly over the pan, then sprinkle using the cheddar. Work the cheese in - off the edges of the pan. Sprinkle with oregano.
3. Spread the marinara sauce around the melting cheese, trying not to work it down into the cheese - rather over it.
4. Add the pepperoni and mushrooms.
5. When the base is golden brown, crispy, and begins to lift as one piece, your pizza is ready.
6. Carefully slide the pizza onto a chopping board or cutting surface and slice into eight equal pieces before serving.

NUTRITION: Calories: 73 Total Fat: 23gCarbs: 1g Protein: 19g

3. .Flatbread Keto Pizza Recipe

Preparation time: 13 minutes Cooking time: 30 minutesServings: 6

INGREDIENTS:
- Almond flour (2.25 cups)
- Coconut flour (2 tablespoons)
- Baking powder (.5 teaspoon)
- Large eggs (3)
- Olive oil (2 tablespoons)
- Salt (.5 teaspoon)
- Pepper (.5 teaspoon)
- Italian seasoning (1 teaspoon)

DIRECTIONS:
1. Warm the oven to 350º Fahrenheit. Use a round - medium pizza pan and cover with parchment baking paper.
2. Sift the baking powder with the almond and coconut flour in a large mixing bowl.
3. In another small container, whisk the eggs and olive oil until you have a frothy texture. Combine the egg mixture into the flour mixture and knead to form a dough ball. Place it in the pan. Top with another sheet of parchment paper and roll out the dough until it is about 0.25-inch thick. Peel off the top piece of parchment paper.
4. Slide the crust with the bottom parchment onto the prepared baking sheet or pizza pan.
5. Bake it until the edges are crispy (partially baked - 15 minutes).
6. Add the chosen toppings with the sauce going on first, then layering cheese, and lastly - the other toppings. Return it to the oven
7. Bake for another 15 minutes until the cheese has melted to your liking.
8. Transfer to the countertop and cool for a couple of minutes.
9. Slice it and serve.

NUTRITION: Calories: 81 Total Fat: 27g Carbs: 5g Protein: 12g

4. .Cheese Crust Pizza

Preparation time: 10 minutes Cooking time: 25 minutesServings: 2
INGREDIENTS:
- 1 28-oz can unsweetened, peeled tomato
- ¼ cup extra-virgin olive oil
- 1 tbsp red wine vinegar
- 1 tsp dried oregano
- 1 tsp dried basil
- 1 tsp dried parsley
- 1 tsp garlic powder
- ½ tsp red pepper flakes
- ¼ tsp black pepper
- salt to taste
- 6 oz shredded mozzarella cheese
- 5 oz cheese of your choice
- 34 medium eggs
- 1 ½ oz pepperoni
- 1 tsp dried oregano

DIRECTIONS:
1. Preheat the oven to 400 F and prepare an oven tray with baking paper or extra-virgin olive oil.
2. To begin your sauce, pour the peeled tomatoes, ½ cup of the tomato liquid, and olive oil into a blender and puree. Add the vinegar, oregano, basil, parsley, garlic powder, red pepper flakes, black pepper, and salt and mix well. Adjust the ingredients to taste.
3. Pour into a sealable container and keep refrigerated.
4. Mix the eggs and 6 oz mozzarella in a bowl and stir well. Place your pizza base on the oven tray, either forming two medium pizzas or 1 large pizza.
5. Bake the crust for 10 minutes. Remove from the oven and let cool for 2 to 3 minutes. Increase the oven temperature to 450 F.
6. Spread about 3 tbsp of tomato sauce over the crust and sprinkle with dried oregano. Add the pepperoni and cheese.
7. Bake for 5 to 10 minutes, making sure the cheese gets a chance to melt and brown to your liking.
8. Serve as is or with a side salad.

NUTRITION: Calories: 1043 Total Fat: 90g Carbs: 5g Protein: 53g

5. Alternate Crust Pepperoni Pizza

Preparation time: 10 minutes Cooking time: 20 minutes Servings: 6

INGREDIENTS:
- 3 ½ cups shredded mozzarella
- 2 tbsp cream cheese
- ¾ cup almond flour
- 1 large egg
- ¼ cup pepperoni
- ⅓ cup unsweetened tomato sauce
- 1 tsp Italian herb mix

DIRECTIONS:
1. Preheat the oven to 425 F and prepare a large pizza pan or oven tray with extra-virgin olive oil or baking paper.
2. In a microwave-safe bowl, mix 2 cups mozzarella and the cream cheese. Microwave on HIGH for 1 ½ minutes. Stir every 30 seconds to ensure the mozzarella melts completely.
3. Add the almond flour, egg, and herb mix, and stir until the ingredients are combined and a dough forms.
4. Place the dough between two sheets of baking paper and roll it out in a 12 inch circle. Remove the baking paper and place the dough in your baking tray.
5. Bake the crust for 10 minutes. Remove from the oven and spread the tomato sauce evenly over the crust. Add the remaining 1 ½ cup mozzarella cheese and pepperoni.
6. Bake for another 10 minutes until the cheese melts and browns. Remove from the oven and let cool for 5 minutes before serving.

NUTRITION: Calories: 235 Total Fat: 19g Carbs: 4g Protein: 18g

6. .Vegetarian Pizza

Preparation time: 15 minutes Cooking time: 35 minutesServings: 6

INGREDIENTS:
- 8 oz shredded mozzarella
- 4 oz cream cheese
- 4 oz of 4 different types of shredded cheese to your taste
- 1 large egg
- ⅓ cup coconut flour
- ⅓ cup almond flour
- ⅓ cup ground golden flax
- 1 big handful baby spinach
- ½ small sliced onion
- 1 tsp minced garlic

DIRECTIONS:
1. Preheat the oven to 400 F. Prepare a pizza pan or oven tray with baking paper or extra-virgin olive oil.
2. In a microwave-safe bowl, mix the mozzarella and 2 oz cream cheese and microwave on HIGH for 1 ½ minutes. Stir every 30 seconds.
3. Stir in the egg, coconut flour, almond flour, and golden flax. Stir until well combined, then knead for 2 to 5 minutes until a uniform, slightly sticky dough forms.
4. Using either your hands or a rolling pin, push the dough evenly into your pizza pan or baking tray. Bake for 20 minutes.
5. While the base bakes, fry the onion in a frying pan over medium heat with a little extra-virgin olive oil for 5 minutes, or until the onion softens and begins to brown. Add the spinach and cover the pan with a lid. Let the mixture cook until the spinach begins to wilt. Remove the frying pan from the heat and set aside to cool.
6. Slightly soften the remaining 2 oz cream cheese in the microwave for a few seconds and mix well with the minced garlic. Spread evenly over the pizza crust once it is done baking.
7. Top the pizza with the spinach mixture and the 4 oz mixed cheese. Bake for another 10 to 15 minutes until the cheese melts and begins to bubble.

NUTRITION: Calories: 383 Total Fat: 29g Carbs: 10g Protein: 18g

7. .Sausage Crust Pizza

Preparation time: 10 minutes Cooking time: 15 minutesServings: 6

INGREDIENTS:
- Sausage – 1 lb.
- Diced onion - 0.5 of 1 small
- Diced red bell pepper - 1
- Sautéed mushrooms – 3 oz.
- Tomato paste – 1 tbsp.
- Mozzarella cheese – 3 oz.
- Sliced ham – 2 oz.
- Onion powder – 1 tsp.
- Garlic powder – 1 tsp.
- Italian seasoning – 1 tsp.
- Also Needed: Medium cake pan

DIRECTIONS:
1. Warm up the oven until it reaches 350ºF.
2. Break the sausage apart and smash onto the sides and bottom of the pan.
3. Once loaded, arrange the pan in the heated oven.
4. Bake for 10 to 15 minutes. Transfer it to a platter when done.
5. Combine the garlic powder, tomato paste, Italian seasoning, onion powder, and garlic powder. Sprinkle over the crust.
6. Note: If you choose, you can store the crust in the freezer until ready to prepare if it will be more than a day before you are prepared to use the crust.
7. To prepare, just layer with the ham, onions, mushrooms, and red pepper. Give it a sprinkle of the mozzarella cheese.
8. Cook for 12 to 15 minutes until golden and the cheese is melted.
9. Store in the refrigerator for a couple of days, but no longer. It is best to freeze as soon as it is cooled.

NUTRITION: Calories: 357 Total Fat: 21.2g Carbs: 12g Protein: 31.3g

8. .Thin Crust White Pizza

Preparation time: 10 minutes Cooking time: 10 minutesServings: 4

INGREDIENTS:
- Grated parmesan cheese - .5 cup
- Egg white protein powder - Unflavored - .25 cup
- Pink Himalayan sea salt – .25 tsp.
- Almond flour - .5 cup
- Large egg - 1
- Heavy whipping cream - 1 tbsp.
- Cream cheese - 2 tbsp.
- Onion or garlic powder – 1 tsp.
- Hard goat cheese - your favorite – .5 cup
- Feta cheese – Crumbled - .33 cup
- Red onion – 1 small
- Seedless Kalamata olives - .25 cup
- Olive oil - 1 tbsp.

DIRECTIONS:
1. Set the temperature of the oven to 400ºF. Line an iron skillet or a cookie sheet with a piece of parchment paper.
2. Whisk each of the dry fixings in a mixing dish. Blend in the egg - mixing by hand. Empty the batter into the baking pan, spreading evenly. Bake for 10-15 min.
3. Prepare the white sauce by mixing the onion/garlic powder, cream cheese, and cream until well combined.
4. Slice the onion. Grate the hard cheese and crumble the feta. You can also chop the olives.
5. Remove the crust when browned and add the white sauce, the cheeses, olives, and onion.
6. Bake 10 minutes or until golden brown. Transfer to the countertop and slice into quarters. Top with some lettuce leaves with a drizzle of the olive oil..

NUTRITION: Calories: 352 Total Fat: 28.9g Carbs: 4.6g Protein: 20g

9. .StLouis-Style Pizza

Preparation time: 10 minutes Cooking time: 10 minutesServings: 6

INGREDIENTS:
- 1/3 cup pizza sauce
- 1/2 cup shredded white cheddar cheese
- 1/4 cup shredded smoked provolone
- 1/4 cup shredded Swiss cheese
- 1 teaspoon dried Italian or pizza seasoning
- 4 bacon strips
- 1/2 thinly sliced onion
- 1/2 thinly sliced seeded bell pepper

DIRECTIONS:
1. Cook cream cheese keto crust as stated above.
2. Remove crust from the oven and increase oven temperature to 450°F.
3. Spread baked keto crust with pizza sauce.
4. Top with bacon strips, onion, and bell pepper.
5. Mix the cheeses and sprinkle with Italian herbs or pizza seasoning.
6. Bake until cheese is melted (from 5 to 10 minutes). Serve.

NUTRITION: Calories: 350.9 Total Fat: 28.3g Carbs: 4.4g Protein: 20.3g

10..New-York style pizza

Preparation time: 10 minutes Cooking time: 10 minutesServings: 6
INGREDIENTS:
- 1/2 cup pizza sauce
- 2 ¼ cup shredded mozzarella
- 1/2 cup grated parmesan cheese
- 2 garlic cloves, minced
- 1 teaspoon dried oregano
- 1 teaspoon red pepper flakes or optional

DIRECTIONS:
1. Cook cream cheese keto crust as stated above.
2. Remove crust from the oven and increase oven temperature to 450°F.
3. Spread pizza sauce on baked keto crust.
4. Sprinkle with garlic, dried oregano, mozzarella and Parmesan cheese, and red pepper flakes.
5. Bake until cheese is melted. Slice and serve immediately.

NUTRITION: Calories: 314.4 Total Fat: 24.3g Carbs: 4.7g Protein: 20g

11..New Haven-Style Clam Pizza

Preparation time: 10 minutes Cooking time: 10 minutesServings: 6
INGREDIENTS:
- 1/2 cup grated Pecorino Romano
- 2 garlic cloves, minced
- 1/8 cup extra-virgin olive oil
- 12 littleneck clams, shucked, cooked
- 1 teaspoon dried oregano, crumbled 1/4 TSP of pink salt
- 1 TSP baking powder—gluten-free
- 1 TSP of oregano (optional)

DIRECTIONS:
1. Mix garlic and oil. Cover the mixture and chill.
2. Cook cream cheese keto crust as stated above.
3. While crust is cooking, let garlic oil come to room temperature.
4. Remove crust from the oven and increase oven temperature to 450°F.
5. Brush dough evenly with garlic oil. Arrange clams over garlic oil and sprinkle with oregano and Romano.
6. Bake about for 10 minutes until cheese is melted, slice and serve hot.

NUTRITION: Calories: 357.7 Total Fat: 28g Carbs: 4.6g Protein: 21.2g

12..Greece-style Pizza

Preparation time: 10 minutes Cooking time: 15 minutesServings: 6

INGREDIENTS:
- 2 teaspoons olive oil
- 1 cup shredded mozzarella
- 1 (6 ounces) bag prewashed baby spinach
- 3/4 cup pizza sauce
- 1 cup crumbled feta cheese
- 1/2 teaspoon ground pepper
- 1 (2 1/4-ounce) can black olives, sliced and drained
- 1 teaspoon dried oregano

DIRECTIONS:
1. Cook spinach in an oiled nonstick skillet over medium-high heat for 3 minutes or until lightly wilted.
2. Cook cream cheese keto crust as stated above.
3. Remove crust from the oven and increase oven temperature to 450°F.
4. Spread baked keto crust with pizza sauce, dried oregano, and mozzarella.
5. Top with cooked spinach, feta cheese, pepper, and olives.
6. Bake until cheese is melted. Serve and enjoy!

NUTRITION: Calories: 263.4 Total Fat: 21.5g Carbs: 5.3g Protein: 12.8g

13..Vegan Bacon Fat Head Pizza

Preparation Time: 35 minutes Servings: 4
INGREDIENTS:
- 1 ½ cups + 2 cups grated mozzarella cheese
- 2 tbsp cream cheese, room temperature
- 2 eggs, beaten
- 1/3 cup almond flour
- 1 tsp dried oregano
- ½ cup sliced vegan bacon

DIRECTIONS:
1. Preheat the oven to 425 F and line a round pizza pan with parchment paper.
2. Combine 1 ½ cups of the mozzarella cheese and dairy* free cream cheese in a safe-microwave bowl and melt in the microwave for 1 minute.
3. Remove from the oven and mix in the eggs and almond flour. Transfer the mixture onto a clean flat surface and knead until smooth.
4. Spread the dough on the pizza pan and bake in the oven for 6 minutes or until golden brown and crusty.
5. Remove from the oven, top with the remaining mozzarella cheese, oregano, and vegan bacon slices.
6. Bake further in the oven for 15 minutes or until the cheese melts.
7. Remove the pizza, slice and serve.

NUTRITION: Calories: 865, Total Fat: 80.2g, Saturated Fat:56.8 g, Total Carbs:19 g, Dietary Fiber:5g, Sugar: 5g, Protein: 28g, Sodium: 1775mg

14..Mushroom-Basil Pizza

Preparation Time: 40 minutes Servings: 4

INGREDIENTS:
- For the crust:
- 1 lb mushroom
- 1 tsp Italian seasoning
- ½ cup grated mozzarella cheese
- ¼ tsp salt
- For the topping:
- ⅔ cup sugar-free tomato sauce
- 1 cup grated mozzarella cheese
- ½ cup fresh basil leaves

DIRECTIONS:
1. Preheat the oven to 425 F and line a pizza pan with parchment paper.
2. In a medium bowl, mix the mushroom, Italian seasoning, mozzarella cheese, and salt until well combined.
3. Spread the mixture on the pizza pan and bake in the oven until the mushroom is cooked and crusty, 18 minutes.
4. Remove from the oven and spread the tomato sauce on top. Scatter the mozzarella cheese on top and then the basil.
5. Bake further for 15 minutes or until the cheese melts.
6. Remove from the oven, slice and serve warm.

NUTRITION: Calories:232 , Total Fat:14.3g, Saturated Fat: 5.4g, Total Carbs: 12 g, Dietary Fiber:4g, Sugar: 4g, Protein:20 g, Sodium:719 mg

15..BBQ Tempeh Pizza

Preparation Time: 40 minutes Servings: 4
INGREDIENTS:
For the crust:
- 1 lb tempeh
- 1 cup grated mozzarella cheese
- 2 eggs, beaten
- ¼ tsp salt

For topping:
- ¼ cup sugar-free BBQ sauce
- 1 ½ cups grated Gruyere cheese
- ¼ cup sliced red onion
- 2 vegan bacon slices, chopped
- 2 tbsp chopped parsley

DIRECTIONS:
1. Preheat the oven to 425 F and line a pizza pan with parchment paper.
2. In a medium bowl, mix the tempeh, mozzarella cheese, eggs, and salt.
3. Spread the mixture on the pizza pan and bake in the oven for 20 minutes or until the tempeh cooks and is crusty.
4. Remove the crust from the oven and spread the BBQ sauce on top. Scatter the Gruyere cheese on top, followed by the red onion, and vegan bacon slices.
5. Bake in the oven for 15 minutes or until the cheese has melted and the back is crispy.
6. Remove the pizza from the oven, slice and serve warm sprinkled with parsley.

NUTRITION: Calories: 341, Total Fat: 30.6g, Saturated Fat:12.3 g, Total Carbs: 8g, Dietary Fiber:2g, Sugar:4 g, Protein:5 g, Sodium: 37mg

16..Tofu & Vegan Bacon Ranch Pizza

Preparation Time: 45 minutes Servings: 4 minutes

INGREDIENTS:

For the crust:
- 2 cups shredded mozzarella cheese
- 2 tbsp cream cheese
- ¾ cup almond flour
- 2 tbsp almond meal

For the ranch sauce:
- 1 tbsp butter
- 2 garlic cloves, minced
- 1 tbsp cream cheese
- ¼ cup coconut cream
- 1 tbsp dry Ranch seasoning mix

For the topping:
- 3 vegan bacon slices, chopped
- 2 tofu
- Salt and black pepper to taste
- 1 cup grated mozzarella cheese
- 6 fresh basil leaves

DIRECTIONS:

1. Preheat the oven to 425 F and line a pizza pan with parchment paper.
2. In a medium safe-microwave bowl, combine the mozzarella and cream cheese. Melt in the microwave for 30 seconds to 1 minute.
3. Remove the bowl from the oven and mix in the almond flour and almond meal.
4. Spread the mixture on the pizza pan and bake in the oven for 15 minutes or until crusty.
5. Meanwhile, in a medium, mix the sauce's ingredientsbutter, garlic, dairy- free cream cheese, coconut cream, and ranch mix. Set aside.
6. Heat a grill pan over medium heat and cook the vegan bacon until crispy and brown, 5 minutes. Transfer to a plate and set aside.
7. Season the tofu with salt, black pepper and grill in the pan on both sides until golden brown and cooked within, 10 minutes. Remove to a plate, allow cooling and cut into thin slices.
8. Spread the ranch sauce on the pizza crust, followed by the tofu and vegan bacon, and then, mozzarella cheese and basil.
9. Bake in the oven for 5 minutes or until the cheese melts.
10. Remove from the oven, slice and serve warm.
11. **NUTRITION:**
12. Calories:339 , Total Fat:34.2 g, Saturated Fat: 18.6g, Total Carbs: 10g, Dietary Fiber:0g, Sugar: 2g, Protein:17 g, Sodium: 283mg

17..Kale-Artichoke Pizza

Preparation Time: 45 minutes Servings: 4

INGREDIENTS:

For the crust:
- 1 ½ cups grated mozzarella cheese
- 2 tbsp cashew cream
- 1 egg, beaten
- 1 tsp Italian seasoning
- ½ tsp garlic powder
- ½ cup almond flour

For the topping:
- 4 tbsp dairy- free cream cheese, room temperature
- ½ cup chopped kale
- ¼ cup chopped artichoke
- 1 lemon, juiced
- ½ tsp garlic powder
- ¼ cup grated parmesan cheese
- ½ cup grated mozzarella cheese
- Salt and black pepper to taste

DIRECTIONS:

1. Preheat the oven to 425 F and line a pizza pan with parchment paper.
2. In a medium safe-microwave bowl, combine the mozzarella and dairy- free cream cheese. Melt in the microwave for 30 seconds to 1 minute.
3. Remove the bowl from the oven and mix in the egg, Italian seasoning, garlic powder, and almond flour.
4. Spread the mixture on the pizza pan and bake in the oven for 15 minutes or until crusty.
5. Remove the crust from the oven and set aside to cool.
6. In a medium bowl, mix the cashew cream, kale, artichoke, lemon juice, garlic powder, parmesan cheese, veganmozzarella cheese, salt, and black pepper.
7. Spread the mixture on the crust and bake again for 15 minutes or slightly golden.

NUTRITION: Calories: 355, Total Fat: 29.9g, Saturated Fat: 12.5g, Total Carbs: 4 g, Dietary Fiber:0g, Sugar:1 g, Protein:18 g, Sodium:324 mg

18..Tomato-Vegan Bacon Pizza

Preparation Time: 45 minutes Servings: 4
INGREDIENTS:
For the crust:
- 1 ½ cups grated mozzarella cheese
- 2 tbsp cream cheese
- ½ cup almond meal
- 1 egg, beaten

For the topping:
- ⅓ cup sugar-free tomato sauce
- ⅓ cup sliced mozzarella
- 4 vegan bacon slices, cut into thirds
- 7 fresh basil leaves, to serve

DIRECTIONS:
1. Preheat the oven to 425 F and line a pizza pan with parchment paper.
2. In a medium safe-microwave bowl, combine the mozzarella and cream cheese. Melt in the microwave for 30 seconds to 1 minute.
3. Remove the bowl from the oven and mix in the almond meal and egg.
4. Spread the mixture on the pizza pan and bake in the oven for 15 minutes or until crusty.
5. Remove the crust from the oven and set aside to cool.
6. Spread the tomato sauce on the crust. Arrange the mozzarella slices on the sauce and then the vegan bacon.
7. Bake again for 15 minutes or until the cheese melts.
8. Remove from the oven and top with the basil. Slice and serve warm.

NUTRITION: Calories: 181, Total Fat: 17.5g, Saturated Fat:11 g, Total Carbs: 6g, Dietary Fiber:3g, Sugar:2 g, Protein: 3g, Sodium: 140mg

19..Mushroom-Pepper Pizza

Preparation Time: 45 minutes Servings: 4
INGREDIENTS:
For the crust:
- 1 ½ cups grated mozzarella cheese
- 2 tbsp dairy- free cream cheese, room temperature
- 1 ½ lb mushroom, crumbled
- ¼ cup coconut flour
- 1 cup almond flour
- ¼ cup grated parmesan cheese
- 2 eggs

For the topping:
- 1 tbsp olive oil
- 1 onion, thinly sliced
- 1 cup chopped mixed bell peppers
- 2 garlic cloves, minced
- 1 cup baby spinach
- ½ cup sugar-free pizza sauce
- 2 cups grated mozzarella cheese
- ½ cup grated cheddar cheese

DIRECTIONS:
1. Preheat the oven to 425 F and line a pizza pan with parchment paper.
2. In a medium safe-microwave bowl, combine the mozzarella and dairy- free cream cheese. Melt in the microwave for 30 seconds to 1 minute.
3. Remove the bowl from the oven and mix in the mushroom, coconut flour, almond flour, parmesan cheese, and eggs.
4. Spread the mixture on the pizza pan and bake in the oven for 15 minutes or until crusty.
5. Remove from the oven and set aside to cool for 2 minutes.
6. Meanwhile, heat the olive oil in a medium skillet and sauté the onion and bell peppers until softened, 5 minutes. Mix in the garlic and cook until fragrant, 30 seconds.
7. Stir in the spinach and allow wilting for 3 minutes. Turn the heat off.
8. Spread the pizza sauce on the crust and top with the bell pepper mixture. Scatter the mozzarella and cheddar cheeses on top.
9. Bake in the oven for 5 minutes or until the cheese melts.
10. Remove from the oven, slice, and serve warm.

Nutrition: Calories:303 , Total Fat: 28.8g, Saturated Fat: 4.2g, Total Carbs: 8 g, Dietary Fiber:4g, Sugar:25 g, Protein: g, Sodium:47 mg

20..Vegetarian Spinach-Olive Pizza

Preparation Time: 40 minutes Servings: 4
INGREDIENTS:
For the crust:
- ½ cup almond flour
- ¼ tsp salt
- 2 tbsp ground psyllium husk
- 1 tbsp olive oil
- 1 cup lukewarm water

For the topping:
- ½ cup sugar-free tomato sauce
- ½ cup baby spinach
- 1 cup grated mozzarella cheese
- 1 tsp dried oregano
- 3 tbsp sliced black olives

DIRECTIONS:
1. Preheat the oven to 425 F and line a baking sheet with parchment paper.
2. In a medium bowl, mix the almond flour, salt, psyllium powder, olive oil, and water until dough forms.
3. Spread the mixture on the pizza pan and bake in the oven until crusty, 10 minutes.
4. When ready, remove the crust and spread the tomato sauce on top.
5. Add the spinach, mozzarella cheese, oregano, and olives.
6. Bake until the cheese melts, 15 minutes.
7. Take out of the oven, slice and serve warm.

Nutrition: Calories: 452, Total Fat: 38.3, Saturated Fat:19.5 g, Total Carbs: 6 g, Dietary Fiber:1g, Sugar: 2g, Protein: 23g, Sodium:746 mg

21..Cauliflower-Vegan Bacon Pizza Casserole

Preparation Time: 40 minutes Servings: 4

INGREDIENTS:
- 4 cups cauliflower rice
- 1 cup grated mozzarella cheese
- 1 tbsp dried thyme
- Salt and black pepper to taste

For the topping:
- ¼ cup sugar-free tomato sauce
- 1 cup grated mozzarella cheese
- ½ cup vegan bacon slices

DIRECTIONS:
1. Preheat the oven to 425 F and lightly grease a baking dish with cooking spray. Set aside.
2. Pour the cauliflower rice in a safe microwave bowl, mix in 1 tablespoon of water and steam in the microwave for 1 minute.
3. Remove the bowl and mix in the mozzarella cheese, thyme, salt, and black pepper. Pour the mixture into the baking dish, spread out and bake in the oven for 5 minutes.
4. Take the dish out of the oven and spread the tomato sauce on top. Scatter the mozzarella cheese on the sauce and then arrange the vegan bacon slices on top.
5. Bake in the oven for 15 more minutes or until the cheese melts.
6. Remove the dish and serve the pizza casserole warm.

Nutrition: Calories: 248, Total Fat: 22.7g, Saturated Fat: 1g, Total Carbs: 5 g, Dietary Fiber:3g, Sugar: 1g, Protein:9 g, Sodium: 227mg

22..Italian Mushroom Pizza

Preparation Time: 45 minutes Servings: 4
INGREDIENTS:
For the crust:
- 1 ½ cups grated mozzarella cheese
- 2 tbsp dairy- free cream cheese
- ½ cup almond meal
- 1 egg, beaten

For the topping:
- 1 tsp olive oil
- 2 medium cremini mushrooms, sliced
- 1 garlic clove, minced
- ½ cup sugar-free tomato sauce
- 1 tsp erythritol
- 1 bay leaf
- 1 tsp dried oregano
- 1tsp dried basil
- 1/2 tsp paprika
- Salt and black pepper to taste
- ½ cup grated mozzarella cheese
- ½ cup grated parmesan cheese
- 6 black olives, pitted and sliced

DIRECTIONS:
1. Preheat the oven to 425 F and line a pizza pan with parchment paper.
2. In a medium safe-microwave bowl, combine the mozzarella and cream cheese. Melt in the microwave for 30 seconds to 1 minute.
3. Remove the bowl from the oven and mix in the almond meal and egg.
4. Spread the mixture on the pizza pan and bake in the oven for 5 minutes or until crusty.
5. Remove the crust from the oven and set aside to cool.
6. Meanwhile, heat the olive oil in a medium skillet and sauté the mushrooms until softened, 5 minutes. Stir in the garlic and cook until fragrant, 30 seconds.
7. Mix in the tomato sauce, erythritol, bay leaf, oregano, basil, paprika, salt, and black pepper. Cook for 2 minutes and turn the heat off.
8. Spread the sauce on the crust, top with the mozzarella and parmesan cheeses, and then, the olives.
9. Bake in the oven until the cheese's melts, 15 minutes.
10. Remove the pizza, slice and serve warm.

NUTRITION: Calories: 452, Total Fat: 38.2g, Saturated Fat: 19.5g, Total Carbs:6 g, Dietary Fiber:1g, Sugar:2 g, Protein: 23g, Sodium: 746mg

23..Extra Cheesy Pizza

Preparation Time: 35 minutes Servings: 4
INGREDIENTS:
For the crust:
- ½ cup almond flour
- ¼ tsp salt
- 2 tbsp ground psyllium husk
- 1 tbsp olive oil
- 1 cup lukewarm water

For the topping:
- ½ cup sugar-free pizza sauce
- 1 cup sliced mozzarella cheese
- 1 cup grated mozzarella cheese
- 3 tbsp grated Parmesan cheese
- 2 tsp Italian seasoning

DIRECTIONS:
1. Preheat the oven to 425 F and line a baking sheet with parchment paper.
2. In a medium bowl, mix the almond flour, salt, psyllium powder, olive oil, and lukewarm water until dough forms.
3. Spread the mixture on the pizza pan and bake in the oven until crusty, 10 minutes.
4. When ready, remove the crust and spread the pizza sauce on top. Add the sliced mozzarella, vegan grated mozzarella, parmesan cheese, and Italian seasoning.
5. Bake in the oven for 18 minutes or until the cheeses melt.
6. Remove from the oven, slice and serve warm.

NUTRITION: Calories: 122, Total Fat: 9.9g, Saturated Fat: 1.3g, Total Carbs: 3 g, Dietary Fiber1:g, Sugar: 1g, Protein: 6g, Sodium:201 mg

24..Spicy and Smoky Pizza

Preparation Time: 45 minutes Servings: 4
INGREDIENTS:
For the crust:
- 2 cups shredded mozzarella cheese
- 2 tbsp dairy- free cream cheese
- ¾ cup almond flour
- 2 tbsp almond meal

For the topping:
- 1 tbsp olive oil
- 1 cup sliced vegan bacon
- ¼ cup sugar-free marinara sauce
- 1 cup sliced smoked mozzarella cheese
- 1 jalapeño pepper, deseeded and sliced
- ¼ red onion, thinly sliced

DIRECTIONS:
1. Preheat the oven to 425 F and line a pizza pan with parchment paper.
2. In a medium safe-microwave bowl, combine the mozzarella and dairy- free cream cheese. Melt in the microwave for 30 seconds to 1 minute.
3. Remove the bowl from the oven and mix in the almond flour and almond meal.
4. Spread the mixture on the pizza pan and bake in the oven for 10 minutes or until crusty.
5. Remove the crust from the oven and set aside to cool.
6. Meanwhile, heat the olive oil and cook the vegan bacon until brown, 5 minutes.
7. Spread the marinara sauce on the crust, top with the mozzarella cheese, vegan bacon, jalapeño pepper, and onion.
8. Bake in the oven until the cheese melts, 15 minutes.
9. Remove from the oven, slice and serve warm.

NUTRITION: Calories:579 , Total Fat: 55.8g, Saturated Fat: 11.4g, Total Carbs: 5g, Dietary Fiber:1g, Sugar: 1g, Protein:6 g, Sodium:452 mg

25..Taco pizza

Preparation Time: 45 minutes Servings: 4 minutes

INGREDIENTS:

For the crust:
- 2 cups shredded mozzarella
- 2 tbsp cream cheese
- 1 egg
- ¾ cup almond flour

For the topping:
- 1 lb mushroom
- 2 tsp taco seasoning
- Salt and black pepper to taste
- ½ cup cheese sauce
- 1 cup grated cheddar cheese
- 1 cup chopped lettuce
- 1 tomato, diced
- ¼ cup sliced black olives
- 1 cup vegan sour cream for topping

DIRECTIONS:
1. Preheat the oven to 425 F and line a pizza pan with parchment paper.
2. In a medium safe-microwave bowl, combine the mozzarella and cream cheese. Melt in the microwave for 30 seconds to 1 minute.
3. Remove the bowl from the oven and mix in the egg and almond flour.
4. Spread the mixture on the pizza pan and bake in the oven for 15 minutes or until crusty.
5. Remove the crust from the oven and set aside to cool.
6. Meanwhile, put the mushroom in a medium pot and cook until brown, 5 minutes. Stir in the taco seasoning, salt, and black pepper.
7. Spread the cheese sauce on the crust and top with the mushroom. Add the cheddar cheese, lettuce, tomato, and black olives.
8. Bake in the oven until the cheese melts, 5 minutes.
9. Remove the pizza from the oven, drizzle the vegan sour cream on top, slice, and serve warm.

NUTRITION: Calories:439 , Total Fat: 31.9g, Saturated Fat:12.2 g, Total Carbs: 9 g, Dietary Fiber:4g, Sugar: 1g, Protein: 36g, Sodium: 574mg

26..Broccoli-Pepper Pizza

Preparation Time: 25 minutes Servings: 4
INGREDIENTS:
For the crust:
- ½ cup almond flour
- ¼ tsp salt
- 2 tbsp ground psyllium husk
- 1 tbsp olive oil
- 1 cup lukewarm water

For the topping:
- 1 tbsp olive oil
- 1 cup sliced fresh mushrooms
- 1 white onion, thinly sliced
- 3 cups broccoli florets
- 4 garlic cloves, minced
- ½ cup sugar-free pizza sauce
- 4 tomatoes, sliced
- ¼ cup chopped basil
- 1 ½ cup grated mozzarella cheese
- ⅓ cup grated parmesan cheese

DIRECTIONS:
1. Preheat the oven to 425 F and line a baking sheet with parchment paper.
2. In a medium bowl, mix the almond flour, salt, psyllium powder, olive oil, and lukewarm water until dough forms.
3. Spread the mixture on the pizza pan and bake in the oven until crusty, 10 minutes.
4. When ready, remove the crust and allow cooling.
5. Heat the olive oil in a medium skillet and sauté the mushrooms, onion, and broccoli until softened, 5 minutes. Mix in the garlic and cook until fragrant, 30 seconds.
6. Spread the pizza sauce on the crust and top with the broccoli mixture, tomato, basil, mozzarella cheese and parmesan cheese.
7. Bake in the oven until the cheeses melt, 5 minutes.
8. Remove from the oven, slice and serve warm.

NUTRITION: Calories:446 , Total Fat: 26.3g, Saturated Fat:12.9 g, Total Carbs: 13g, Dietary Fiber:3g, Sugar:7 g, Protein:42 g, Sodium: 1101mg

27..Caramelized Onion and Ricotta cheese Pizza

Preparation Time: 35 minutes Servings: 4
INGREDIENTS:
For the crust:
- 2 cups grated mozzarella cheese
- 2 tbsp dairy- free cream cheese, room temperature
- 2 large eggs, beaten
- ⅓ cup almond flour
- 1 tsp dried Italian seasoning

For the topping:
- 2 tbsp butter
- 2 red onions, thinly sliced
- Salt and black pepper to taste
- 1 cup crumbled ricotta cheese
- 1 tbs almond milk
- 1 cup fresh curly endive, chopped

DIRECTIONS:
1. Preheat the oven to 425 F and line a round pizza pan with parchment paper.
2. Combine the mozzarella cheese and dairy- free cream cheese in a safe-microwave bowl and melt in the microwave for 1 minute.
3. Remove from the oven and mix in the eggs, almond flour, and Italian seasoning.
4. Spread the dough on the pizza pan and bake in the oven for 6 minutes or until golden brown and crusty.
5. Meanwhile, melt the butter in a large skillet and stir in the onions. Reduce the heat to low, season the onions with salt, black pepper, and cook with frequent stirring until caramelized, 15 to 20 minutes. Turn the heat.
6. In a medium bowl, mix the ricotta cheese with the almond milk and spread on the crust. Top with the caramelized onions.
7. Bake in the oven for 10 minutes and take out after.
8. Top with the curly endive, slice the pizza and serve warm.

NUTRITION: Calories:131 , Total Fat:10.5 g, Saturated Fat: 4.3g, Total Carbs: 3g, Dietary Fiber:1g, Sugar: 1g, Protein:7 g, Sodium: 375mg

28..Tofu Scampi Pizza

Preparation Time: 35 minutes Servings: 4

INGREDIENTS:

For the crust:
- ½ cup almond flour
- ¼ tsp salt
- 2 tbsp ground psyllium husk
- 1 tbsp olive oil
- 1 cup lukewarm water

For the topping:
- 2 tbsp butter
- 2 tbsp olive oil
- 2 garlic cloves, minced
- ¼ cup white wine
- ½ tsp dried basil
- ½ tsp dried parsley
- ½ lemon, juiced
- ½ lb chopped tofu
- 2 cups grated cheese blend
- ½ tsp Italian seasoning
- ¼ cup grated parmesan cheese

DIRECTIONS:
1. Preheat the oven to 425 F and line a baking sheet with parchment paper.
2. In a medium bowl, mix the almond flour, salt, psyllium powder, olive oil, and lukewarm water until dough forms.
3. Spread the mixture on the pizza pan and bake in the oven until crusty, 10 minutes.
4. When ready, remove the crust and allow cooling.
5. Meanwhile, heat the butter and olive oil in a medium skillet. Sauté the garlic until fragrant, 30 seconds.
6. Mix in the white wine, allow reduction by half and stir in the basil, parsley, and lemon juice. Cook for 1 minute and stir in the tofu. Cook for 3 minutes or until pink and opaque.
7. Stir in the cheese blend and Italian seasoning. Allow cheese melting, 3 minutes. Turn the heat off.
8. Spread the tofu mixture on the crust and top with the parmesan cheese. Bake for 5 minutes or until the parmesan cheese has melted.
9. Remove the pizza from the oven, slice and serve warm.

NUTRITION: Calories:217 , Total Fat: 14.2g, Saturated Fat:7.5 g, Total Carbs: 9 g, Dietary Fiber:3g, Sugar:4 g, Protein: 15g, Sodium: 401mg

29..Strawberry-Tomato Pizza

Preparation Time: 35 minutes Servings: 4
INGREDIENTS:
For the crust:
- 2 cups shredded mozzarella cheese
- 2 tbsp cream cheese
- ¾ cup almond flour
- 2 tbsp almond meal

For the topping:
- 1 cup grated mozzarella cheese
- 2 celery stalks, chopped
- 1 medium tomato, chopped
- 1 tbsp olive oil
- Salt and black pepper to taste
- 2 tbsp balsamic vinegar, divided
- 1 cup fresh strawberries, halved
- 1 tbsp chopped mint leaves

DIRECTIONS:
1. Preheat the oven to 425 F and line a pizza pan with parchment paper.
2. In a medium safe-microwave bowl, combine the mozzarella and cream cheese. Melt in the microwave for 30 seconds to 1 minute.
3. Remove the bowl from the oven and mix in the almond flour and almond meal.
4. Spread the mixture on the pizza pan and bake in the oven for 10 minutes or until crusty.
5. Remove the crust from the oven and set aside to cool.
6. Spread the mozzarella cheese on the crust.
7. In a medium bowl, toss the celery and tomato with the olive oil, salt, black pepper, and balsamic vinegar. Spoon the mixture onto the mozzarella cheese and arrange the strawberries on top. Top with the mint leaves.
8. Bake in the oven until the cheese melts, 15 minutes.
9. Remove the pizza from the oven, slice and serve warm.

NUTRITION: Calories:556 , Total Fat:44g, Saturated Fat: 26g, Total Carbs: 11 g, Dietary Fiber:2g, Sugar:7 g, Protein: 31g, Sodium: 1235mg

30..Mediterranean Pizza

Preparation Time: 30 minutes Servings: 4
INGREDIENTS:
For the crust:
- ½ cup almond flour
- ¼ tsp salt
- 2 tbsp ground psyllium husk
- 1 tbsp olive oil
- 1 cup lukewarm water

For the topping:
- ¼ tsp red chili flakes
- ¼ tsp dried Italian seasoning
- 1 cup crumbled cottage cheese
- 3 sliced plum tomatoes
- 6 pitted Kalamata olives, chopped
- 5 basil leaves, chopped for garnishing

DIRECTIONS:
1. Preheat the oven to 425 F and line a baking sheet with parchment paper.
2. In a medium bowl, mix the almond flour, salt, psyllium powder, olive oil, and lukewarm water until dough forms.
3. Spread the mixture on the pizza pan and bake in the oven until crusty, 10 minutes.
4. When ready, remove the crust and allow cooling.
5. Sprinkle the red chili flakes and Italian seasoning on the crust and top with the cottage cheese.
6. Use the back of a spoon to press the cheese onto the crust and arrange the tomatoes and olives on top.
7. Bake in the oven for 10 to 12 minutes and remove afterwards.
8. Garnish the pizza with the basil, slice and serve warm.

NUTRITION: Calories: 438, Total Fat: 32g, Saturated Fat:18 g, Total Carbs: 10g, Dietary Fiber:2g, Sugar:5 g, Protein: 30g, Sodium: 771mg

31..Pesto Arugula Pizza

Preparation Time: 30 minutes Servings: 4

INGREDIENTS:

For the crust:
- ½ cup almond flour
- ¼ tsp salt
- 2 tbsp ground psyllium husk
- 1 tbsp olive oil
- 1 cup lukewarm water

For the topping:
- 1 cup basil pesto, olive oil-based
- 1 cup grated mozzarella cheese
- 1 tomato, thinly sliced
- 1 zucchini, cut into half-moon pieces
- 1 cup baby arugula
- 2 tbsp chopped pecans
- ¼ tsp red chili flakes

DIRECTIONS:

1. Preheat the oven to 425 F and line a baking sheet with parchment paper.
2. In a medium bowl, mix the almond flour, salt, psyllium powder, olive oil, and lukewarm water until dough forms.
3. Spread the mixture on the pizza pan and bake in the oven until crusty, 10 minutes.
4. When ready, remove the crust and allow cooling.
5. Spread the pesto on the crust and top with the mozzarella cheese, tomato, and zucchini.
6. Bake in the oven until the cheese melts, 15 minutes.
7. Remove the pizza from the oven; top with the arugula, pecans, and red chili flakes.
8. Slice and serve the pizza warm.

NUTRITION: Calories:253 , Total Fat: 18.8g, Saturated Fat:7,8 g, Total Carbs: 9 g, Dietary Fiber:2g, Sugar:2 g, Protein: 14g, Sodium: 583mg

32..Four Cheese Mexican Pizza

Preparation Time: 30 minutes Servings: 4

INGREDIENTS:

For the crust:
- 2 cups shredded mozzarella cheese
- 2 tbsp cream cheese
- ¾ cup almond flour
- 2 eggs, beaten

For the topping:
- ¾ lb mushroom
- 2 tsp taco seasoning mix
- Salt and black pepper to taste
- ½ cup vegetable broth
- 1 ½ cups salsa
- 2 cups of melted mozzarella cheese

DIRECTIONS:
1. Preheat the oven to 425 F and line a pizza pan with parchment paper.
2. In a medium safe-microwave bowl, combine the mozzarella and cream cheese. Melt in the microwave for 30 seconds to 1 minute.
3. Remove the bowl from the oven and mix in the almond flour and eggs.
4. Spread the mixture on the pizza pan and bake in the oven for 15 minutes or until crusty.
5. Remove the crust from the oven and set aside to cool.
6. Add the mushroom to a medium pot and cook until brown, 5 minutes. Stir in the taco seasoning, salt, black pepper and vegetable broth. Cook for 3 minutes or until thickened. Stir in the salsa.
7. Spread the mixture onto the crust and scatter the cheese blend on top.
8. Bake further in the oven until the cheese melts, 15 minutes.
9. Remove the pizza, slice and serve warm

NUTRITION: Calories: 390, Total Fat: 29.3g, Saturated Fat:17.2 g, Total Carbs: 7g, Dietary Fiber:1g, Sugar:2 g, Protein: 25g, Sodium: 609mg

33..Chicago style thin-crust Pizza

Preparation time: 10 minutes Cooking time: 20 minutesServings: 6
INGREDIENTS:
- 4 oz. pepperoni
- 1 cup ground pork
- 2 jalapeños, sliced thinly
- 2 oz. sliced mushrooms
- 1 thinly sliced onion
- 1/2 teaspoon fennel seeds, crushed
- 3/4 cup pizza sauce
- 1/2 cup each of Smoked Provolone, Swiss and White Cheddar, grated and blended
- 1/8 cup extra-virgin olive oil
- 1 teaspoon dried oregano

DIRECTIONS:
1. In a large nonstick skillet cook jalapeños, onion, and mushrooms with 2 teaspoons of oil for 7-10 minutes over medium-high heat. Remove to cool.
2. Roast the ground pork and add the oil, fennel, and salt and pepper (to taste).
3. Cook cream cheese keto crust as stated above.
4. Remove crust from the oven and increase oven temperature to 450°F.
5. Spread baked keto crust with pizza sauce, dried oregano, the pepperoni, and cheese.
6. Top with the ground pork, onion, jalapeños, and mushrooms.
7. Bake about 12 minutes or until cheese is melted. Cool for 10 minutes, and then slice and enjoy!

NUTRITION: Calories: 322.9 Total Fat: 26.9gCarbs: 4.3g Protein: 15.8g

34..Regina Pizza

Preparation time: 10 minutes Cooking time: 10 minutes Servings: 6

INGREDIENTS:
- 1/3 cup your favorite pizza sauce
- 2 cups thinly sliced fresh mushrooms
- 1 1/2 cups chopped ham
- 2 cups shredded mozzarella cheese
- 1 sliced tomato
- 1 ounce sliced black olives, drained
- 1 teaspoon dried oregano

DIRECTIONS:
1. Place sliced mushrooms in a small microwave-safe bowl. Microwave on high power until mushrooms are tender (for 2 to 3 minutes). Drain mushrooms.
2. Cook cream cheese keto crust as stated above.
3. Remove crust from the oven and increase oven temperature to 450°F.
4. Spread baked keto crust with pizza sauce and sprinkle with oregano.
5. Add the tomato, mozzarella, ham, mushrooms, and olives.
6. Bake until cheese is melted. Serve hot.

NUTRITION: Calories: 275.1 Total Fat: 21.6g Carbs: 2.6g Protein: 18.1g

35..Margherita Pizza

Preparation time: 10 minutes Cooking time: 15 minutesServings: 6

INGREDIENTS:
- 1 tablespoon olive oil
- 2 cloves garlic, finely chopped
- 1/4 cup pizza sauce
- 8 oz. mozzarella cheese
- 2 tomatoes, sliced
- fresh basil
- fresh ground pepper, to taste

DIRECTIONS:
1. Combine the olive oil and chopped garlic in a small dish.
2. Cook cream cheese keto crust as stated above.
3. Remove crust from the oven and increase oven temperature to 450°F.
4. Spread baked keto crust with olive oil/garlic mixture.
5. Top with pizza sauce, mozzarella cheese slices, and tomato slices.
6. Bake until cheese is melted. Remove from the oven. Top with basil and pepper before serving.

NUTRITION: Calories: 288.6Total Fat: 23.3gCarbs: 4.8gProtein: 15.7g

36..Marinara Pizza

Preparation time: 10 minutes Cooking time: 10 minutesServings: 6

INGREDIENTS:
- 2 tablespoons olive oil
- 3 cloves garlic, finely chopped
- 1/3 cup your favorite pizza sauce
- 1 1/2 cup mozzarella cheese, grated
- 100 g cherry tomatoes, halved
- 1/2 cup cooked salmon, chopped
- 1 ounce sliced black olives, drained
- 1 teaspoon dried oregano
- handful of fresh basil

DIRECTIONS:
1. Mix olive oil and chopped garlic in a small dish.
2. Cook cream cheese keto crust as stated above.
3. Remove crust from the oven and increase oven temperature to 450°F.
4. Spread baked keto crust with olive oil/garlic mixture.
5. Spread tomato sauce, dried oregano, cherry tomatoes, salmon, and sliced black olives.
6. Top with mozzarella cheese and fresh basil.
7. Bake for 5 to 10 minutes until cheese is melted. Serve and enjoy!

NUTRITION: Calories: 383.5 Total Fat: 31.3g Carbs: 5.8g Protein: 20.5g

37..Napoli Pizza with Anchovies

Preparation time: 10 minutes Cooking time: 15 minutesServings: 6

INGREDIENTS:
- 2/3 cup pizza sauce
- 1 tablespoon olive oil
- 1 1/2 cups shredded mozzarella cheese
- 6 to 8 small anchovies
- 1 tablespoon salted capers, rinsed
- 1 teaspoon dried oregano
- pinch chili flakes (optional)

DIRECTIONS:
1. Cook cream cheese keto crust as stated above.
2. Remove crust from the oven and increase oven temperature to 450°F.
3. Spread baked keto crust with olive oil and pizza sauce, leaving a 1-inch border.
4. Scatter the mozzarella cheese over pizza.
5. Arrange the anchovies and capers.
6. Sprinkle the oregano and chili flakes (if using) over the pizza.
7. Bake until cheese is melted. Slice and enjoy!

NUTRITION: Calories: 303.3 Total Fat: 24.7g Carbs: 4.2g Protein: 16.8g

38..Capricciosa Pizza

Preparation time: 10 minutes Cooking time: 15 minutesServings: 6

INGREDIENTS:
- 1/2 cup puréed tomatoes (passata)
- white mushrooms in oil (champignons)
- 7 green olives, pitted
- 7 black olives, pitted
- 3 artichoke hearts, quartered
- 1 cup mozzarella cheese, shredded
- 1 tablespoon olive oil
- Salt to taste
- 1 teaspoon dried oregano

DIRECTIONS:
1. Prepare tomato sauce by mixing puréed tomatoes with olive oil, dried oregano, and salt.
2. Cook cream cheese keto crust.
3. Remove crust from the oven and increase oven temperature to 450°F.
4. Spread baked keto crust with tomato sauce.
5. Arrange olives, mushrooms, artichokes, and mozzarella cheese over the pizza.
6. Place the pizza in the oven for 10 minutes until cheese is melted. Serve and enjoy!.

NUTRITION: Calories: 317.9 Total Fat: 27.1g Carbs: 5.8g Protein: 14g

39..Pizza Frittata

Preparation time: 15 minutes Cooking time: 30 minutesServings: 8

INGREDIENTS:
- 12 eggs
- 9 ounce bag frozen spinach
- 1 ounce pepperoni
- 5 ounces mozzarella cheese
- 1 teaspoon garlic, minced
- ½ cup ricotta cheese
- ½ cup parmesan cheese,
- 4 tablespoon olive oil
- 1/4 teaspoon nutmeg
- Salt
- Pepper

DIRECTIONS:
1. Microwave the spinach on defrost.
2. Preheat your oven to 375°F.
3. Combine the ricotta, the parmesan and spinach.
4. Pour the mixture into a baking dish.
5. Sprinkle the mozzarella over the mixture.
6. Add the pepperoni.
7. Bake for half an hour, until set.Place the pizza back into the oven for 2 to 3 minutes to heat the toppings.

NUTRITION: Calories: 298 Total Fat: 23.8g Carbs: 2.1g Protein: 19.4g

40..Keto Gluten-Free Pizza Crust

Preparation time: 10 minutes Cooking time: 5 minutesServings: 6

INGREDIENTS:
1. 3 ounces of almond flour
2. 2 teaspoons of xanthan gum
3. 2 teaspoons of apple cider vinegar
4. 5 teaspoons of water
5. 1 ounce of coconut flour
6. 1 egg
7. ¼ teaspoon of salt
8. 2 teaspoons of baking powder
9. Marinara sauce
10. Fresh basil
11. Salami
12. Pepperoni
13. Green Peppers
14. Onions
15. Mozzarella cheese
16. Mushrooms

DIRECTIONS:
1. Combine the almond flour, baking powder, coconut flour, xanthan gum, and salt into a large bowl. Mix well. You can also use a food processor.
2. While you are still stirring the mixture (or the food processor is running on pulse) you will slowly add the apple cider vinegar. Mix well.
3. Crack the egg into a small bowl and whisk well.
4. Pour the egg into the mixture.
5. Pour in the water immediately after the egg.
6. Mix all the ingredients until the dough starts to form into a ball.
7. Because the dough is sticky, wrap it in plastic wrap before you start kneading.
8. If you start to notice the dough is cracking, place it back into your food processor or bowl and mix in more water. Only add in one teaspoon of water at the time. Continue this process until the dough has no more than a couple of cracks.
9. Allow the dough to sit at room temperature for 10 minutes.
10. Place a skillet on high heat.
11. While the skillet is heating up, place the dough between two sheets of parchment paper and roll out the dough to make the pizza crust. Depending on how thick you want the crust will determine how wide the dough is.
12. Wet your fingertips and press down on the side of the dough.
13. Place your pizza crust in the pan and cook on both sides. It should take 2-3 minutes but might be a bit longer. You want the crust to blister.
14. When you flip over your pizza crust, add your toppings.
15. Serve and enjoy!

NUTRITION: Calories: 118 Total Fat: 9g Carbs: 6g Protein: 5g

41..Personal Pan Pizza Crusts

Preparation time: 10 minutes Cooking time: 7 minutesServings: 6

INGREDIENTS:
- ½ cup of almond flour
- 8 egg whites, best to use large eggs
- ½ teaspoon of baking powder
- Your choices of seasonings. However, the best seasonings are pepper, parsley, Italian seasoning, and salt.
- If you want a thicker crust, you will use 3 egg whites and 5 whole eggs. If you want a thinner crust, use 8 egg whites. It's best to use large eggs.
- ½ teaspoon of baking powder
- ¼ cup of sifted coconut flour
- Your choices of seasonings. However, be best are salt, Italian seasoning and salt. Many people also like to sift extra coconut flour to create a flour dusting on the pizza crust.
- 2 cloves of crushed garlic
- 1 teaspoon of dried basil
- ½ cup of Mutti tomato sauce
- ¼ teaspoon of sea salt

DIRECTIONS:
1. In a large mixing bowl, add in the eggs. Whisk well.
2. Sift your chosen flour into the eggs. Combine until all the clumps are removed from the mixture.
3. Combine the baking powder and your chosen seasonings. Mix well.
4. Place a small pan on low heat.
5. Lightly grease the pan with oil, butter, or cooking spray.
6. Add batter into the pan once it is hot. You want to ensure your pan is hot or the batter won't turn out correctly.
7. Cover your pan for 3 to 4 minutes.
8. Once you start to notice bubbles at the top of your crust, flip the crust over to cook the other side. You shouldn't have to cook the second side for very long. You want to watch the crust carefully as it will burn quickly.
9. Continue cooking the batter until it is gone.
10. Set the pizza crusts on the side to continue cooling. You want to make sure they are completely cooled before you add any toppings.
11. In a medium-sized bowl, add the tomato sauce, sea salt, garlic, and basil. Mix well.
12. Allow the sauce to sit at room temperature for at least 30 minutes. This will allow it to thicken.
13. Pour onto the pizza crusts and then add your additional toppings, such as mozzarella cheese, salami, pepperoni, mushrooms, and green peppers.

NUTRITION: Calories: 198 Total Fat: 1g Carbs: 6g Protein: 8g

42..Egg and Gluten-Free Pizza

Preparation time: 15 minutes Cooking time: 30 minutesServings: 6

INGREDIENTS:
- 2 tablespoons cream cheese, full-fat
- ½ teaspoon of salt
- 8 ounces of mozzarella cheese, full-fat
- 1/3 cup of almond flour
- 2 tablespoons grated parmesan cheese
- 2 tablespoons of whole or ground psyllium husk
- ½ teaspoon of garlic powder

DIRECTIONS:
1. Preheat your oven to 425 degrees Fahrenheit.
2. Shred the mozzarella cheese into a microwavable container.
3. Place the cheese in the microwave and heat for one minute.
4. Stir the cheese and place back into the microwave for another 30 seconds.
5. Remove the cheese from the microwave and let it cool for 30 seconds to one minute.
6. Combine the cream cheese, parmesan, almond flour, salt, and garlic powder. Mix well. You will find it helpful to knead the dough with your hands for a couple of minutes when mixing.
7. Add the psyllium husk into the mixture. Combine well.
8. Place a piece of parchment paper on a flat surface.
9. Roll the dough into a ball and place on the parchment paper.
10. Set another piece of parchment paper on top of the dough.
11. Roll out the dough with a rolling pin until it is at least a quarter-inch thick.
12. Shape the dough as you would like.
13. Remove and discard the top piece of parchment paper.
14. Transfer the bottom piece of parchment paper and dough onto your pizza pan.
15. Place the pizza crust into the oven and bake for 15 to 20 minutes.
16. Remove the pizza from the oven, flip the crust, and place it back into the oven for five minutes.
17. Remove the pizza and add the pizza sauce and your favorite toppings.
18. Place the pizza back in the oven to back for another five minutes.
19. Once the pizza is done, remove it from the oven and allow it to cool for 5 to 10 minutes before you cut.
20. Serve and enjoy!

NUTRITION: Calories: 161Total Fat: 13gCarbs: 2g Protein: 9g

43..Pizza Ball Head

Preparation time: 10 minutes Cooking time: 12 minutesServings: 6
INGREDIENTS:
- 5½ oz. mozzarella cheese, grated
- ¾ cup of almond flour
- 2 tablespoons cream cheese
- 1 C. White wine vinegar
- An egg
- ½ c. Salt tea
- Olive oil to grease your hands
- 8 oz fresh Italian sausage
- 1 tbsp. Butter
- ½ cup unsweetened tomato sauce
- ½ c. Dried oregano
- 4½ oz. mozzarella cheese, grated

DIRECTIONS:
1. Preheat oven to 400 ° F (200 ° C).
2. Heat mozzarella and including the cream cheese in a small nonstick skillet over medium heat or in a microwave-safe bowl.
3. Stir until they are melted. Add all the ingredients and mix well.
4. Moisten your hands with a some olive oil and flatten the dough on baking paper forming a circle of 18 cm (7 in) in diameter. Use the rolling pin to flatten the dough between two sheets of parchment paper.
5. Remove the top parchment leaf. Prick the crust with a fork and bake for 10-15 minutes until golden brown.
6. Remove it from the oven.
7. While the crust is still cooking, sauté the sausage meat in the olive oil.
8. Spread a small layer of tomato sauce over the crust. Garnish the pizza with meat and cheese. Bake for about 10 to 12 minutes until cheese is melted.
9. Sprinkle with oregano and serve with a green salad.

NUTRITION: Calories: 154 Total Fat: 27g Carbs: 10g Protein: 17g

44..Keto Pizza with Chicken and Garlic

Preparation time: 10 minutes Cooking time: 15 minutesServings: 6
INGREDIENTS:
- 6 large eggs, egg white and egg yolk separated
- ½ teaspoon tartar
- 6 tbsp neutral egg white powder or (if tolerable) neutral whey protein powder
- 90 g double cream cheese (if tolerated), room warm, or the above 6 egg yolks, lightly whisked
- 3 slices of bacon, diced
- 1 small onion, diced
- 2 chicken thighs, meat loosened from the bones and cut into 1 cm cubes
- 240 ml tomato sauce
- 60 ml of coconut aminos or gluten-free tamari sauce
- 5 tbsp erythritol or ½ tsp liquid stevia extract
- 60 ml of coconut vinegar
- 1 roasted garlic bulb, toes raised, or 3 raw garlic cloves, crushed with the knife blade
- 2 tsp liquid smoke
- 110 g Provolone or Cheddar (if tolerated), grated

DIRECTIONS:
1. Preheat your oven at 160 ° C. Then grease a lasagna shape (about 37 × 28 cm) or a cast-iron pan (diameter about 30 cm).
2. For the dough, place the egg whites and tartar in a bowl and beat very stiff with the hand mixer (or place in the blender and let the appliance run for about 5 minutes). Set the appliance to the lowest setting and mix in the egg white or whey protein powder. Carefully fold in the cream cheese or the yolks with a spatula.
3. Fill the dough into the pan or pan and spread with a uniformly thick layer. Put in the oven and bake for 18 minutes.
4. Meanwhile, for the toppings and the sauce, place bacon and onions in a large pan and fry until the bacon becomes crispy. Add the meat cubes and sauté for 5 minutes. Remove bacon, onions and meat with a sifting spoon and place in a bowl. Put aside.
5. Leave the fat in the pan. Add the tomato sauce, coconut aminos or tamari sauce, erythritol or stevia extract, vinegar, garlic and liquid smoke and stir thoroughly. Add the mixture to the blender and puree to a smooth sauce.
6. Remove the pizza base from the oven and heat to 200 ° C. increase.
7. Spread the sauce, bacon-meat mixture and cheese evenly on the pizza base. Bake the keto pizza in the oven for another 5 minutes until the cheese is melted and slightly browned. Serve warm.

NUTRITION: Calories: 617 Total Fat: 42g Carbs: 5.2gProtein: 51.8g

45..High-protein Pizza Cabbage with Nutri-plus

Preparation time: 10 minutes Cooking time: 10 minutesServings: 6

INGREDIENTS:
- 200 gspelt flour
- 60mlNutri-Plus Protein Powder Neutral
- 200 ml of water
- 10mlbaking powder
- 100 ml Sieved tomatoes
- 1 tbsp. mixed herbs
- 80mlcolorful paprika
- 30mlmushrooms
- 30mlpeas
- 20mlolives
- 1 spring onion
- SmoothingSalt, pepper, paprika

DIRECTIONS:
1. Preheat the oven to 180 ° C.
2. Put the spilled flour, the protein powder, the baking powder and a pinch of salt in a bowl and mix everything thoroughly.
3. Now add the water and knead the mass into a firm dough.
4. Divide the dough into 4 pieces to form flat baguettes.
5. Place the baguettes on the baking sheet lined and the baking paper and bake for about 5 minutes.
6. In time you take care of the surface. Mix the tomato with herbs and spices and cut the vegetables into small cubes.
7. Remove the pre-baked baguettes from the oven, sprinkle with the tomato sauce and spread the toppings on top.
8. Bake the pizza cabbies for another 10 minutes until they are nicely brown and crispy.

NUTRITION: Calories: 265 Total Fat: 2g Carbs: 40g Protein: 20g

46..Pulled Pork with Pineapple

Preparation time: 10 minutes Cooking time: 8 hours | Serving: 6

INGREDIENTS:
- Roast pork shoulder
- Pork shoulder roast 1.5 kg (3 1/3 lb), with bone
- Pineapple cut into small cubes 1 box of 398 ml, with the juice
- Apple cider vinegar 45 ml (3 tablespoons)
- Tomato paste 1 box of 156 ml
- Brown sugar 45 ml (3 tablespoons)

DIRECTIONS:
1. In a skillet, heat a little olive oil over medium heat. Sear the roast pork 1 minute on all sides.
2. Place the diced pineapples with their juice, cider vinegar, tomato paste, brown sugar, onion and, if desired, the steak seasoning in the slow cooker — season with salt, peppers, and mix.
3. Place the shoulder roast in the slow cooker and flip it over several times to coat with sauce. Cover and cook for 8 hours at low intensity.
4. Remove the roast from the cooker and let cool on a plate.
5. Pour the slow cooker sauce into a saucepan. Boil, and then simmer over low-medium heat until the sauce has reduced by half.
6. Fray the roast with two forks, and then add the meat to the pan and stir.

NUTRITION: Calories: 657 Total Fat: 36g Carbs: 31g Protein: 52g

PASTA RECIPES
47..Creamy Zoodles

Preparation time: 2 minutes Cooking time: 3 minutes Servings: 1

INGREDIENTS:
- Three (3) cloves of mincedgarlic
- Two (2) tablespoons of butter
- Two (2) medium zucchini
- A quarter teaspoon salt to taste
- A quarter teaspoon pepper
- A quarter cup of parmesan cheese

DIRECTIONS:
1. Wash your zucchini then cut it to strands using a spiralizer or vegetable peeler then set aside. If done right, your zucchini should come out like spaghetti strands. I mean, that's the point right?
2. Put a large pan on medium heat. Put the butter in to melt and then add minced garlic. Stir fry the garlic until it starts to appear translucent. If you know you have an affinity for burning things, please be attentive so the garlic doesn't get burnt.
3. Add your zucchini strands and stir fry for three minutes. Make sure to taste your noodle strands to check how tender they are as zucchini cooks really fast. Try not to "taste" till it finishes.
4. Bring down the pan, add salt, pepper and parmesan cheese, stir until well combined and serve..

NUTRITION: Calories: 100 Total Fat: 4g Carbs: 4g Protein: 4g

48..Keto Ricotta Gnocchi

Preparation time: 15 minutes Cooking time: 45 minutes Servings: 2
INGREDIENTS:
- One large egg yolk
- A quarter cup of butter
- One large egg
- A half cup of Mozzarella cheese
- Half a cup of almond flour
- A teaspoon of lemon zest
- A quarter cup ofsalted butter
- A teaspoon of fresh thyme leaves

DIRECTIONS:
1. Put butter and mozzarella cheese into a medium bowl and microwave for a minute.
2. Stir the mixture and microwave for another minute.
3. Let mixture cool for 2-3 minutes.
4. Stir in almond flour, egg yolk and egg.
5. Stir until dough starts to come together.
6. Coat a smooth surface with some almond flour and knead dough until it becomes stretchy and smooth (If the dough is too sticky, add a teaspoon of almond flour and knead until it comes together).
7. Use your hand to roll up the dough, as if trying to shape a long rolling pin. It should be at least a half inch wide and an inch in diameter. Then cut into small bite sizes. You can cut them into any shape you want. If you have an artistic side you can cut them into little stars or bow ties.
8. Freeze the gnocchi for 20 minutes or until you are ready to eat them.
9. When you are ready, add some salt to a pot of water and set to boil on medium heat. Be careful not to let the water boil too much or the gnocchi will break apart.
10. Set the gnocchi to boil for 2-3 minutes or until it starts to float on the surface of the water.
11. Remove the gnocchi and set to drain in a sieve or paper lined plate and let cook for a few minutes.
12. Put the butter to melt in a large pan on medium heat.
13. Add thyme and lemon zest and cook for 1-2 minutes.
14. Add the cooked gnocchi, stir and let cook for 2 minutes.
15. Season with pepper and salt or as desired.

NUTRITION: Calories: 250 Total Fat: 19g Carbs: 5g Protein: 14g

49..Keto Carbonara Pasta

Preparation time: 10 minutes Cooking time: 15 minutes Servings: 1

INGREDIENTS:
- 150 grams of bacon
- One large egg yolk
- A packet of miracle noodles
- A cup of heavy whipping cream
- Two (2) tablespoons of parmesan cheese
- 60 grams of chicken breast

DIRECTIONS:
1. Dice the chicken and Chicken in separate plates.
2. Set both to cook separately in a frying pan for 5 minutes.
3. Note: Do not let the bacon become crispy.
4. Put parmesan cheese and egg yolk in a small bowl and mix until it forms a paste.
5. Pour the cheese mixture into a frying pan and put on medium heat.
6. Add half the amount of cream and mix until a smooth creamy paste is formed.
7. Add the other half of the cream, bacon and chicken. Stir until fully coated.
8. Dry fry miracle noodles in another pan for 10 minutes, stirring continuously so it doesn't stick or burn.
9. Mix the noodles with sauce and serve.

NUTRITION: Calories: 580 Total Fat: 50g Carbs: 5g Protein: 27g

50..Fresh Egg Pasta

Preparation time: 40 minutes Cooking time: 25 minutes Servings: 1

INGREDIENTS
- One large egg yolk
- A cup of low moisture Mozzarella cheese (shredded)

DIRECTIONS
1. Put the mozzarella into a point and microwave for 1-2 minutes
2. Take the cheese out and stir until fully melted. If cheese appears to have lumps, microwave for 1 more minute.
3. Let cool for 1-3 minutes before adding the egg (to avoid scrambling it).
4. Stir the yolk and cheese mixture until you have a smooth yellow dough.
5. Line a flat surface with a pieceof parchment paper and place your dough on it.
6. Cover the dough with another parchment and use a rolling pin to flatten and thin out. Continue thinning it out until your dough is less than a quarter inch thick.
7. Remove the top parchment and cut your dough into long, thin strips.
8. When you are done,place your strips of dough (with bottom piece of parchment paper) on a flat tray or plate and put into the refrigerator to dry out.
9. Refrigerate overnight or if you are in a hurry, 6-8 hours would do.
10. When you are ready to cook, boil a pot of water on medium heat.
11. Put in the pasta and let cookfor 1 minute. You have to be careful not to overcook if or the pasta will begin to break and melt.
12. Once the pasta is ready, sieve and run under cold water to cool.
13. Use your hands to gently peel apart any strands that might be glued together.

NUTRITION: Calories: 358 Total Fat: 22g Carbs: 3g Protein: 33g

51..Palmini Low-Carb Pasta

Preparation time: 5 minutes Cooking time: 2 minutes Servings: 1

INGREDIENTS:
- A tablespoon of butter
- Two (2) tablespoons of parmesan cheese (shredded)
- Four (4) fresh basil leaves
- A quarter teaspoon of black pepper.
- A can of palmini linguine (drained and rinsed)
- A quarter teaspoon of salt

DIRECTIONS:
1. Boil the drained and rinsed palmini in a pot of water for five minutes on medium heat.
2. Drain the palmini.
3. Put the cheese and butter in a bowl and microwave for 1 minute or until fully melted.
4. Sprinkle some salt on the parmini and pour it into the melted cheese, add pepper and serve with a few leaves of fresh basil.

NUTRITION: Calories: 201 Total Fat: 14g Carbs: 12g Protein: 9g

52..Keto Shirataki Noodles

Preparation time: 2 minutes Cooking time: 3 minutes Servings: 1

INGREDIENTS:
- A tablespoon of unsalted butter
- A quarter cup of grated Parmesan
- A quarter teaspoon of garlic powder
- A quarter teaspoon of Kosher salt
- A quarter teaspoon of black Pepper
- A pack of miracle noodles

DIRECTIONS:
1. Drain and rinse noodles because they tend to have a fishy smell.
2. Put a pot of water to boil on medium heat. Once it starts to boil, put in the noodles and let cook for 2-3 minutes, drain.
3. Put a large pan on medium-low and dry-roast the noodles.
4. Add butter, salt, garlic powder, and pepper. Stir fry.
5. Turn off the heat and put the noodles into a plate.
6. Sprinkle some parmesan cheese and serve.

NUTRITION: Calories: 0 Total Fat: 0g Carbs: 0g Protein: 0g

53..Keto Butter Cabbage Noodles

Preparation time: 5 minutes Cooking time: 10 minutes Servings: 2

INGREDIENTS:
- A quarter cup of unsalted butter
- A teaspoon of dried oregano
- A clove of garlic (diced)
- Half a cup of parmesan cheese (shredded)
- A teaspoon of salt
- A teaspoon of dried basil
- A head of green cabbage
- A quarter cup of red pepper flakes
- Half a bulb of onion

DIRECTIONS:
1. Wash the cabbage and cut into thin long strips then set aside.
2. Dice the onion and garlicthen set aside
3. Melt butter on medium -highin a non-stick frying pan
4. Saute the minced onion and garlic until they start to brown.
5. Add chili flakes, salt and herbs and stir until well combined.
6. Add the cabbage and stir until it is fully coated in the mixture.
7. Cook for 2-3 minutes or until it loses moisture and starts to wilt.
8. Note: If you cook it for too long,it will lose too much moisture and become too soft. We want it to have a spaghetti feel to it, so turn it down when it can perfectly fold around a fork.
9. Put the cabbage in a plate and sprinkle some parmesan cheese on top then serve.
10. You can spice up your cabbage noodles with some diced chicken, bacon or minced beef.

NUTRITION: Calories: 187 Total Fat: 5g Carbs: 1g Protein: 3g

54..Keto Shrimp Scampi

Preparation time: 20 minutes Cooking time: 10 minutes Servings: 1

INGREDIENTS:
- A quarter cup of chicken broth
- A quarter teaspoon of red chili flakes
- A pinch of salt
- One pound of shrimp
- A clove of garlic (minced)
- Two (2) tablespoons of parsley (chopped)
- Two (2) tablespoons of lemon juice
- Two (2) tablespoons of unsalted butter
- Two (2) summer squash

DIRECTIONS:
1. Use a spiralizer or vegetable peeler to cut the summer squash into strands.
2. Sprinkle with salt and spread the noodles on an absorbent piece of parchment or paper towel, set aside for 15 minutes.
3. Use the paper towel to wring out the excess moisture in the noodles.
4. In a non-stick pan, melt butter, and stir fry garlic until it starts to turn brown.
5. Add lemon juice, chicken broth and chili flakes, stir and set on medium-low for 3 minutes.
6. Once it starts to boil, add the shrimp, let boil for another 3 minutes or until shrimps start to turn a light shade of pink, then reduce the heat to low and let it simmer.
7. Taste the sauce and add pepperand salt to your liking.
8. Put in the summer squash noodles and parsley, stirring gently so as to coat the noodles in the sauce.

NUTRITION: Calories: 334 Total Fat: 13.1g Carbs: 8.49g Protein: 48.4g

55..Vietnamese Pasta Bowl

Preparation time: 20 minutes Cooking time: 25 minutes Servings: 1

INGREDIENTS:
- A pinch of salt
- A quarter pounder of shrimp Butterfield
- 25 grams of chopped peanuts
- Half a cup of cucumber
- Four(4) cups of romaine's lettuces (chopped)
- 25 great of pork ribs(thinly cut)
- Two (2) packs of Shirataki noodles (rinsed and drained)
- Nine (9) sprigs of cilantro
- 20 grams of sprouted mung beans
- A pound of boneless country style
- A quarter cup of fish sauce (Red coat)
- Two (2)tablespoons of white rice vinegar
- A quarter cup of water
- Two (2) tablespoons of Erythritol
- A tablespoon spoon of garlic chili sauce

DIRECTIONS:
1. Boil the noodles for 3-5 minutes, then drain.
2. Put the noodles in the fridge until the salad is ready to be served.
3. Sprinkle some salt on shrimps and pork ribs and grill until well cooked, then set aside.
4. Share the already prepared sales ingredients into four different bowls.
5. Note: The bowls should be big enough to stir and toss salad in without spilling.
6. Put the cooked noodles, romaine, cooked shrimp and pork, cilantro, peanuts, cucumber and mung beans.
7. Put fish sauce, white rice vinegar, garlic chili sauce, Erythritol and water in a bowl and mix until well combined.
8. Drizzle a generous amount over your salad, then toss to combine. Serve as desired.

NUTRITION: Calories: 300 Total Fat: 17g Carbs: 4g Protein: 31g

56..Keto Japanese Seafood Pasta

Preparation time: 5 minutes Cooking time: 10 minutes Servings: 2

INGREDIENTS:
- Two (2) cloves of garlic
- Three (3) tablespoons of Heavy cream
- Half an onion(diced)
- Half a cup of Clam juice
- A teaspoon of soy sauce
- A tablespoon of salted butter
- A pack of Shirataki noodles
- A quarter teaspoon of black pepper
- A tablespoon of Kewpie mayo
- Two (2) tablespoons of white wine
- Frozen seafood mix (preferably shrimp, clams and bay scallops)

DIRECTIONS:
1. If your seafood mix is frozen, thaw it until fully melted.
2. Bring water to boil in a medium sized pot.
3. Strain the shirataki noodles to get rid of pre-packed liquid.
4. Run the noodles under cold water, put in a bowl then set aside.
5. Dice the onions and garlic then set aside.
6. Put soy sauce, kewpie mayo, and heavy creaminto a small bowl then mix until fully combined then set aside.
7. Once the water starts to boil, put in the shirataki noodles, and cook for 2-3 minutes (this is mostly to remove the taste of the pre-packedliquid from the noodles)
8. Strain the noodles and set aside.
9. Preheat a large frying pan on medium heat and melt the butter and stir fry onions.
10. Fry onions until it starts to turn brown.
11. Add white wine, seafood mix, clam juice and garlic and cook, stirring until seafood gets completely cooked through and the liquid in the pan dries up.
12. Pour in the sauce from step 5 and reduce the heat to low. Stir the mixture until full combinedand let cook for another minute.
13. Pour the sauce over the shirataki noodles and enjoy!

NUTRITION: Calories: 325 Total Fat: 11g Carbs: 4g Protein: 14g

57..Low carb Spaghetti & Fettuccine

Preparation time: 2 minutes Cooking time: 3 minutes Servings: 1

INGREDIENTS:
- Three (3) cloves of mincedgarlic
- Two (2) tablespoons of butter
- Two (2) medium zucchini
- A quarter teaspoon salt to taste
- A quarter teaspoon pepper
- A quarter cup of parmesan cheese

DIRECTIONS:
1. Wash your zucchini then cut it to strands using a spiralizer or vegetable peeler then set aside. If done right, your zucchini should come out like spaghetti strands. I mean, that's the point right?
2. Put a large pan on medium heat. Put the butter in to melt and then add minced garlic. Stir fry the garlic until it starts to appear translucent. If you know you have an affinity for burning things, please be attentive so the garlic doesn't get burnt.
3. Add your zucchini strands and stir fry for three minutes. Make sure to taste your noodle strands to check how tender they are as zucchini cooks really fast. Try not to "taste" till it finishes.
4. Bring down the pan, add salt, pepper and parmesan cheese, stir until well combined and serve..

NUTRITION: Calories: 100 Total Fat: 4g Carbs: 4g Protein: 4g

58..Low carb fettuccine Alfredo (with Brussel sprouts or roasted broccoli)

Preparation time: 5 minutes Cooking time: 30 minutes Servings: 3

INGREDIENTS:
- 4 tablespoons butter
- 2 tablespoons minced garlic
- 2 cups heavy whipping cream
- 1 block parmesan cheese about 140g
- 1 can Palmini heart of Palm noodles
- Pink Himalayan salt (for taste).

DIRECTIONS:
1. Using a saucepan, melt the butter over medium heat.
2. Add the cream, garlic, and salt and stir.
3. Cut off the rind from the cheese and add to the mixture.
4. Grate the cheese into the saucepan and stir.
5. Minimize the heat to low and let it simmer. (till it attains the consistency you like)
6. Remove the rind and discard.
7. Drain and rinse the Palmini noodles.
8. Add the noodles to the sauce.
9. Remove from the heat and serve.

NUTRITION: Calories: 464 Total Fat: 11g Carbs: 4g Protein: 4g

59..Low carb Lasagna (with cucumber salad or sautéed spinach)

Preparation time: 10 minutes Cooking time: 40 minutes Servings: 6

INGREDIENTS:
- ¼ cup white onion, chopped
- 1 ½ cup Marinara sauce
- 1 cup shredded mozzarella, divided
- 2/3 cup parmesan cheese, divided
- ½ cup Ricotta cheese
- 3/4 teaspoon garlic powder, divided
- 1 teaspoon oregano, divided
- 1 lb. ground beef
- ½ lb. Italian sausage

DIRECTIONS:
1. Preheat your oven to 400ºF
2. Using a cast-iron skillet or pan (should be oven-safe), brown your ground beef and sausage together. Do this over medium heat on your stove which will take about 15 minutes.
3. Add the onion to sauté with the meat. (till the meat softens)
4. Pour in the marinara sauce, adding ½ teaspoon of oregano and ½ teaspoon of garlic powder into the skillet. Let it simmer for 5 minutes.
5. Using a clean bowl, add the ½ cup mozzarella, 1/3 cup Parmesan and the ricotta. Mix these ingredients well before adding the remaining garlic powder and oregano. Add some pepper and salt for taste and fold the mixture till they combine.
6. Turn the stove heat off, evenly spreading the meat in the pan till it creates a uniform layer.
7. Use a spoon to place the cheese mixture around the pan and slightly push them down to the bottom with it.
8. Top with the remaining Parmesan and mozzarella.
9. Bake for 20 minutes (till it turns golden)

NUTRITION: Calories: 514 Total Fat: 15g Carbs: 4.6g Protein: 21g

60..Keto lasagna (with roasted cauliflower or roasted broccoli).

Preparation time: 10 minutes Cooking time: 50 minutes Servings: 4
INGREDIENTS:
- 1 lb. ground beef
- 1 cup marinara sauce
- ¼ cup onion, minced
- 1 cup shredded mozzarella cheese
- 6 tablespoons ricotta cheese
- 1 teaspoon Italian seasoning
- 1 tsp. Italian seasoning
- 4 oz. cream cheese, full fat & softened
  - cups shredded mozzarella cheese
- 2 large eggs

DIRECTIONS:
1. W Preheat your oven to 355ºF
2. Line your baking tray (9 x 13 inch) with parchment paper.
3. Blend all your cheese dough ingredients in a food processor until it has completely mixed. Mixing by hand is possible too if you don't have one. The mixture should have a thick consistency.
4. Slowly pour the batter from the food processor into the baking pan, spreading it uniformly with a spatula.
5. Bake for 20 minutes in the middle section. (The top should be firm when you touch it)
6. Let the cheese noodles cool while you turn your full attention to the next task. (making the meat sauce)
7. Add the onion and ground beef in a skillet over medium heat till they brown.
8. Add the marinara sauce and Italian seasoning and minimize to low heat. Let it simmer for 3 minutes.
9. Now slice cheese dough noodles into thirds. (they should fit into a loaf pan of 8 x 4 inches)
10. In an 8 x 4 loaf pan spread a thin layer of the meat sauce at the bottom. Place the first dough noodle layer over the sauce.
11. Add 1/3 of the meat sauce left, over the first layer, then evenly spread on 3 tablespoons ricotta and ¼ mozzarella cheese.
12. Add the second noodle and repeat the process above. (meat sauce, ricotta then mozzarella)
13. Add the third dough noodle topping it with the remaining meat sauce and mozzarella. You can add a pinch of oregano to it.
14. Bake for 20 minutes in the middle section of your oven at 350ºF
15. Let it bubble and blister for 1 to 2 minutes after the 20 minutes.
16. Let it cool before serving.

NUTRITION: Calories: 633 Total Fat: 11g Carbs: 16g Protein: 30g

61..Fathead low carb gnocchi (with basil pesto or mushroom cream sauce).

Preparation time: 2 minutes Cooking time: 3 minutes Servings: 1
INGREDIENTS:
- Three (3) cloves of mincedgarlic
- Two (2) tablespoons of butter
- Two (2) medium zucchini
- A quarter teaspoon salt to taste
- A quarter teaspoon pepper
- A quarter cup of parmesan cheese

DIRECTIONS:
1. Wash your zucchini then cut it to strands using a spiralizer or vegetable peeler then set aside. If done right, your zucchini should come out like spaghetti strands. I mean, that's the point right?
2. Put a large pan on medium heat. Put the butter in to melt and then add minced garlic. Stir fry the garlic until it starts to appear translucent. If you know you have an affinity for burning things, please be attentive so the garlic doesn't get burnt.
3. Add your zucchini strands and stir fry for three minutes. Make sure to taste your noodle strands to check how tender they are as zucchini cooks really fast. Try not to "taste" till it finishes.
4. Bring down the pan, add salt, pepper and parmesan cheese, stir until well combined and serve..

NUTRITION: Calories: 100 Total Fat: 4g Carbs: 4g Protein: 4g

62..Fathead low carb gnocchi (with basil pesto or mushroom cream sauce).

Preparation time: 10 minutes Cooking time: 25 minutes Servings: 5

INGREDIENTS:
- 2 cups blanched almond flour, very fine
- ¼ cup butter
- 2 cups shredded mozzarella cheese, full fat
- 1 egg yolk, large
- 1 egg, large
- ¼ cup salted butter
- 1 teaspoon fresh thyme leaves
- 1 teaspoon lemon zest

DIRECTIONS:
1. In a bowl (microwave safe) put the mozzarella cheese and butter. Microwave for a minute, remove and stir.
2. Microwave for another minute, remove and stir it vigorously. (till it completely combines) Let it cool for about two minutes.
3. Add in the egg, egg yolk and flour. Mix till dough forms and knead it with your hands on a smooth surface. Add some almond flour if the dough is too wet.
4. Form a long rollout of the dough of about 1-inch diameter. Then, cut the roll into 1/2" wide pieces. Form disks same in shape as the photo above.
5. For 15 minutes freeze the gnocchi before cooking. (this will make them firm)
6. Put the gnocchi in a gentle boil of salted water. (A vigorous one will cause the pieces to fall apart) Boil for 1 to 2 minutes.
7. Slowly remove the gnocchi from the salted water and place them on a paper towel-lined plate.
8. Put them aside and let them cool for 5 minutes.
9. Prepare for the next step. (making the sauce)
10. In a sauté pan, melt the butter.
11. Add the thyme leaves and lemon zest, cooking 2 minutes.
12. Add the gnocchi into the pan and cook for 2 minutes.
13. Season the pasta with pepper and salt.

NUTRITION: Calories: 497 Total Fat: 13g Carbs: 4.9g Protein: 22g

63..Low carb egg pasta

Preparation time: 5 minutes Cooking time: 5 minutes Servings: 2

INGREDIENTS:
- 2 eggs
- 1 ounce cream cheese
- ¼ teaspoon wheat gluten

DIRECTIONS:
1. Preheat your oven to 325ºF
2. In a blender, put the eggs, cream cheese & wheat gluten. (Blend for a minute)
3. Spread the batter on the baking pan.
4. Bake for 5 minutes. (avoid over-baking)
5. Let it cool then cut into the shape you desire.

NUTRITION: Calories: 111 Total Fat: 2g Carbs: 0g Protein: 9g

64..Low carb pasta

Preparation time: 10 minutes Cooking time: 1 minutes Servings: 1
INGREDIENTS:
- 1 cup low moisture mozzarella cheese
- 1 egg yolk, large

DIRECTIONS:
1. In a bowl (microwave-safe), put the cheese. Microwave for a minute, remove and stir. Microwave for another minute or less till the cheese melts.
2. Let the cheese cool to avoid cooking the egg. (not for too long)
3. Add the egg yolk in the bowl of melted cheese and stir. Stir until an even yellow dough form.
4. Place the yellow dough between two pieces of parchment papers and roll it using a rolling pin. (should be 1/8" thick)
5. Omit the top parchment paper.
6. Cut the dough into strips of ½" width. Keep the pasta in your refrigerator for 6 hours.
7. Cook in a pot of water to boil. Do this for 1 minute to avoiding over-cooking. Remove from the pot and drain the water.
8. Let it cool then serve with your favorite sauce.

NUTRITION: Calories: 358 Total Fat: 12g Carbs: 3g Protein: 32g

65..Low carb pasta (with basil pesto);

Preparation time: 10 minutes Cooking time: 10 minutes Servings: 4

INGREDIENTS:
- 1.16oz Parmesan cheese, grated
- 1.31oz mozzarella cheese, grated
- 4 ounces cream cheese, softened
- 1/8 tsp. garlic powder
- 1/8 tsp. ground pepper
- 1/8 tsp. dried marjoram
- 1/8 tsp. ground oregano
- 1/8 tsp. dried basil
- 1/8 tsp. dried tarragon
- 3 egg yolks

DIRECTIONS:
1. Preheat your oven at 475ºF then lower to 350ºF.
2. Beat the egg yolks and cream cheese in a bowl.
3. Add the remaining cheese (Parmesan & mozzarella) into the bowl and beat with a hand mixer.
4. Add all the spices and continue mixing.
5. Line your baking pan with parchment paper.Spread your batter evenly in the pan. (use a spatula)
6. Bake for about 8 minutes while keeping a close eye on it to avoid over-baking. Lower to 300ºF once you notice small bubbles and bake for an additional 2 minutes. (Ensure all sides of the pasta are done)
7. Let it cool for about 15 minutes.
8. Begin slicing in accordance to the shape you desire.

NUTRITION: Calories: 165 Total Fat: 6g Carbs: 1g Protein: 11g

66..Cheese head lasagna sheets

Preparation time: 3 minutes Cooking time: 15 minutes Servings: 8

INGREDIENTS:
- 1 egg
- 2 tbsps. cream cheese
- ¾ cup almond flour
- 1 ¾ cups shredded mozzarella cheese
- ¼ tsp salt
- ½ tsp Italian seasoning

DIRECTIONS:
1. In a microwave safe bowl, mix the shredded cheese and almond flour.
2. Add the cream cheese on top of the mix.
3. Put the mix in the microwave for 30 seconds.
4. Mix in the Italian seasoning, salt, and egg.
5. Shape into a sphere with your hands.
6. Put the ball in in the middle of the two pieces of parchment paper.
7. Roll the dough out into a sheet using a rolling pin.
8. Remove the parchment paper on top.
9. Cut into 4 wide 6-inch-long pieces.
10. Prepare the lasagna sauce and filling.
11. Preheat the oven to 400ºF.
12. Cook for 12-15 minutes.

NUTRITION: Calories: 275 Total Fat: 7.6g Carbs: 1.6g Protein: 6.3g

67..Faux egg noodles

Preparation time: 4 minutes Cooking time: 8 minutes Servings: 1

INGREDIENTS:
- 2 eggs
- 1 oz. cream cheese
- A pinch garlic powder
- A pinch onion powder
- A pinch salt
- A pinch pepper

DIRECTIONS:
1. Preheat oven to 325ºF.
2. In a blender, mix all the ingredients together until the mixture is smooth.
3. Cover the pan with parchment paper and pour the mixture on the paper.
4. Bake for 8 minutes.
5. To prevent further cooking, remove the parchment paper and the pasta from the pan immediately after taking it out of the oven.
6. Roll the slightly cooled pasta and cut into noodles of your desired size.

NUTRITION: Calories: 258 Total Fat: 16g Carbs: 4.8g Protein: 14.7g

68..Stove made Keto Cauliflower Mac and cheese

Preparation time: 15 minutes Cooking time: 30 minutes Servings: 4

INGREDIENTS:
- 1 head cauliflower (separated into florets)
- 3 tablespoons butter (salted)
- 2 teaspoons arrow powder/ ½ teaspoon konjac
- ½ teaspoon Dijon mustard
- ¼ teaspoon black pepper (ground)
- ¼ teaspoon garlic powder
- 1 ½ cups cheddar cheese (shredded & sharp)
- 1 cup heavy cream, Kosher salt to taste.

DIRECTIONS:
1. Using a Dutch oven, brown the butter over medium heat. This will take about 5 minutes.
2. Add your heavy cream, mustard, garlic powder, black pepper and salt into the Dutch oven.
3. Add in the cauliflower and stir, ensuring every piece is coated.
4. Simmer for about 15 minutes. (Till the cauliflower soften)
5. Mix the arrowroot powder/ konjac powder with a few tablespoons of water. Pour this into the Dutch oven and stir. (Till it forms a thick consistency)
6. Add your cheddar cheese and stir. Ensure it completely melts & serve.

NUTRITION: Calories: 323 Total Fat: 11g Carbs: 7g Protein: 12g

69..Kelp noodle salad

Preparation time: 10 minutes Cooking time: 0 minutes Servings: 4

INGREDIENTS:
- 3 green onions (sliced)
- 1 (11oz/340g) pack kelp noodles
- 1 cucumber (julienned)
- ¼ cup carrots (grated)
- ½ cup cashews (crushed)
- 0.5 oz. cilantro (minced)
- 2.3oz almond butter
- 1 garlic clove (minced)
- 1 tablespoon tamari/ coconut aminos
- 1 tablespoon swerve
- 2 tablespoons lime juice
- 1 teaspoon chili oil/ chili infused extra-virgin olive oil
- 1 teaspoon ginger root (grated)
- 1 teaspoon sesame oil
- Red pepper flakes (pinch)
- Sea salt (pinch).

DIRECTIONS:
1. In a bowl mix the salad ingredients.
2. In a jar, mix the dressing ingredients. (seal the jar and shake to mix well)
3. Pour the dressing into the initial bowl.
4. Toss to mix and serve.

NUTRITION: Calories: 240 Total Fat: 11g Carbs: 4.6g Protein: 7g

70..Kelp noodles (with sesame chicken).

Preparation time: 5 minutes Cooking time: 25 minutes Servings: 4
INGREDIENTS:
- 1 lb. chicken breast (cut in pieces),
- 10 oz. mushrooms (sliced)
- E12 oz. kelp noodles
- 2 cup broccoli
- 3 carrots (large in size & chopped)
- 1 teaspoon olive oil
- 2 tablespoons toasted sesame oil
- 3 tablespoon sesame seeds
- 2 cloves garlic (minced)
- 1/3 cup coconut aminos.

DIRECTIONS:
1. In a skillet, heat olive oil over medium heat.
2. Add the mushrooms and fry for about 6 to 8 minutes. (ensure the mushroom liquid has completely evaporated)
3. Include the chicken, broccoli, and carrots. Fry for about 8 minutes.
4. In a bowl, add and whisk all the sauce ingredients.
5. Include the noodles and sauce to the pan. (cook for 5 minutes)
6. Season the dish with sea salt.

NUTRITION: Calories: 394 Total Fat: 10g Carbs: 7g Protein: 29g

71..Palmini noodles (with sausage ragu).

Preparation time: 5 minutes Cooking time: 35 minutes Servings: 4

INGREDIENTS:
- 5 bratwurst sausages, without casings
- 2/3 cup parmesan cheese, grated
- ½ cup parsley, chopped
- ¼ cup Ruby port wine
- 28oz whole tomatoes, peeled
- bay leaves
- 1 carrot, medium in size & grated
- 1 Oregano
- Palmini noodles, 1 can
- 1 tablespoon Fennel seeds
- 2 tablespoons Extra-virgin olive oil, divided
- 2 tablespoons garlic, chopped
- 1 teaspoon red pepper flakes.

DIRECTIONS:
1. Heat up I tablespoon of olive oil in a Dutch oven over medium heat.Add in the fennel seeds and bratwurst, cooking until the sausage begins browns. (takes 5 minutes)
2. Add in the carrot right away and cook with the sausage till it is entirely cooked. (another 5 minutes)
3. Add the remaining tablespoon of olive oil into the Dutch oven.Add in oregano, garlic, and red pepper flakes and cook for about 30 seconds.
4. Pour in the wine, bringing it to a boil. Cook for about 2 minutes till it almost evaporates.
5. Add in the tomatoes and bay leaves. Minimize the heat and simmer for 15 minutes. (Remove the bay leaves)
6. Add in the noodles and combine well.
7. Add in parmesan and parsley, stirring for 3 minutes.
8. Serve.

NUTRITION: Calories: 253 Total Fat: 6g Carbs: 4.7g Protein: 6.9g

72..Butternut squash noodles.

Preparation time: 10 minutes Cooking time: 15 minutes Servings: 4

INGREDIENTS:
- 6 cups Butternut squash noodles, spiralized
- ½ cup walnuts, chopped
- ½ cup parmesan cheese, shredded
- 2 tablespoons Carepelli Extra virgin olive oil
- 1 onion, chopped
- 2 cloves garlic, minced
- ¼ teaspoon black pepper, ground
- Salt to taste

DIRECTIONS:
1. Heat up the oil in a pan over medium heat.
2. Add the onion into the pan and cook for 4 minutes. (till it turns translucent)
3. Add in the garlic, letting it cook before stirring for 30 seconds.
4. Add in the noodles, cooking them for about 10 minutes. They tend to soften and shrink when cooked.
5. Add the walnuts and stir gently.
6. Serve with freshly chopped parsley and parmesan cheese.

NUTRITION: Calories: 408 Total Fat: 7g Carbs: 6g Protein: 5.4g

73..Shirataki noodles (with mushrooms)

Preparation time: 2 minutes Cooking time: 3 minutes Servings: 1
INGREDIENTS:
- Three (3) cloves of mincedgarlic
- Two (2) tablespoons of butter
- Two (2) medium zucchini
- A quarter teaspoon salt to taste
- A quarter teaspoon pepper
- A quarter cup of parmesan cheese

DIRECTIONS:
1. Wash your zucchini then cut it to strands using a spiralizer or vegetable peeler then set aside. If done right, your zucchini should come out like spaghetti strands. I mean, that's the point right?
2. Put a large pan on medium heat. Put the butter in to melt and then add minced garlic. Stir fry the garlic until it starts to appear translucent. If you know you have an affinity for burning things, please be attentive so the garlic doesn't get burnt.
3. Add your zucchini strands and stir fry for three minutes. Make sure to taste your noodle strands to check how tender they are as zucchini cooks really fast. Try not to "taste" till it finishes.
4. Bring down the pan, add salt, pepper and parmesan cheese, stir until well combined and serve..

NUTRITION: Calories: 100 Total Fat: 4g Carbs: 4g Protein: 4g

74..Creamy Zoodles

Preparation time: 10 minutes Cooking time: 15 minutes Servings: 2

INGREDIENTS:
- Shirataki noodles, 2 packages
- 3 cups assorted mushrooms
- Olive oil
- 2 tablespoons butter
- 2 cloves garlic
- Dried parsley, pinch
- 300ml thick cream
- 1 teaspoon almond flour
- ¼ teaspoon pepper
- ¼ teaspoon salt
- Freshly chopped parsley

DIRECTIONS:
1. Rinse and drain the shirataki noodles.
2. Add the noodles into a pan over medium heat for 3 minutes.
3. Remove the noodles from the pan, setting it aside. Heat up butter using the same pan then add garlic.
4. Add the mushrooms in the pan and cook for about 5 minutes. Make sure that the mushrooms are fully coated before removing and setting aside.
5. With the oil residing on the pan, add the dried parsley, almond flour, cream and stir constantly to combine.
6. Add the shirataki noodles and mushrooms back into the pan mix well & season, serve & garnish.

NUTRITION: Calories: 237 Total Fat: 20g Carbs: 4g Protein: 6g

75..Butternut squash noodles (with mushroom cream sauce)

Preparation time: 10 minutes Cooking time: 20 minutes Servings: 4
INGREDIENTS:
- 1 butternut squash, peeled
- 3 sprigs thyme, fresh
- 8 ounces mushrooms, sliced
- 2 tablespoons butter
- 1 cup heavy cream
- ½ cup chicken broth
- Salt & Pepper to taste

DIRECTIONS:
1. Use a spiralizer to spiralize the butternut squash.
2. In a large skillet, heat up butter over medium heat. Add mushrooms, thyme sprigs, pepper & salt. (sauté till mushroom softens)
3. Add the broth and cream then stir.
4. Add the butternut squash and minimize the heat. Cover with a lid and simmer.
5. Season with pepper and salt.

NUTRITION: Calories: 307 Total Fat: 23g Carbs: 6g Protein: 5g

76..Shirataki noodles (with coconut Basil chicken)

Preparation time: 10 minutes Cooking time: 15 minutes Servings: 4
INGREDIENTS:
- 1 lb. raw chicken breast, thinly cut
- 8ounces cucumber
- 10 basil leaves, large
- E1 can coconut milk, full-fat
- 31 tablespoon coconut oil
- Miracle noodles, 2 packages
- E2 tablespoons fish sauce
- 2 tablespoons sweetener
- ¼ cup lime juice
- ½ teaspoon toasted sesame oil
- Sesame seeds
- Toasted coconut, shredded
- Red pepper flakes
- Mint
- Basil
- Cilantro

DIRECTIONS:
1. Cut the chicken into thin strips. In a pan, heat up the coconut oil over medium heat till hot. Add all the chicken strips, sautéing for about 7 minutes. Ensure the pieces are entirely cooked before removing.
2. Ensure you've juiced up a 1/4 cup of lime juice. Add the fish sauce and your sweetener to the cup and stir to mix well. Take out 3 tablespoons of the sauce and add into your blender with a pinch of salt. Add 1/2 teaspoon toasted sesame oil to the blender too.
3. Pee your cucumber and spiralize it with a spiralizer. (You can dice it instead if you lack one)
4. Allow the chicken juice residing on the pan to turn brown and solidify. Add basil leaves and pour in coconut milk while scraping the brown bits. Thereafter, bring it to boil over high heat for 5 minutes. When done, pour it into the blender blending till smooth. (Vent the lid since the liquid is hot)
5. Rinse and drain the noodles. Using a bowl (microwave-safe), heat up the noodles to warm.
6. Add the remaining sweet and sour sauce over the cucumber noodles and toss.
7. Add the sauce and chicken back into the pan. (heat over medium heat till hot)
8. Divide the kelp noodles among 4 bowls.
9. Top the noodles with basil chicken.
10. Garnish the cucumber salad as you wish.

NUTRITION: Calories: 285 Total Fat: 22g Carbs: 5g Protein: 18g

77..Rosemary lasagna noodles

Preparation time: 3 minutes Cooking time: 40 minutes Servings: 4
INGREDIENTS:
- 2 eggs
- 4 oz. cream cheese
- ¼ cup parmesan, shredded
- 1 ¼ cup mozzarella, shredded
- 1/8 tsp rosemary
- pinch of marjoram
- pinch of thyme
- ½ tsp basil
- ½ tsp oregano
- ¼ tsp garlic powder
- ¼ tsp onion powder
- ¼ tsp salt

DIRECTIONS:
1. Preheat the oven to 325ºF.
2. Mix the cream cheese and eggs in a bowl until smooth.
3. Add in the remaining ingredients.
4. Pour the mixture on a baking tray lined with parchment paper.
5. Bake for 25 minutes.
6. Cut the lasagna noodles while the pasta sheet is still warm.
7. Prepare the filling (Meaty Keto Lasagna Filling).
8. Layer the noodles and the filling.
9. Bake for another 20 minutes.
10. Serve while hot.

NUTRITION: Calories: 199 Total Fat: 11g Carbs: 1.9g Protein: 12.7g

78..Baked Zucchini Noodles with Feta

Preparation time: 10 minutes Cooking time: 15 minutes Servings: 3

INGREDIENTS:
- Spiralized zucchini (2)
- Quartered plum tomato (1)
- Feta cheese (8 cubes)
- Pepper and salt (1 teaspoon of each)
- Olive oil (1 tbsp.)

DIRECTIONS:
1. Lightly grease a roasting pan with a spritz of cooking oil.
2. Set the oven temperature at 375º Fahrenheit.
3. Slice the noodles with a spiralizer, and add the olive oil, tomatoes, pepper, and salt.
4. Bake the noodle dish for 10 to 15 minutes. Transfer from the oven and add the cheese cubes, tossing to combine. Serve.

NUTRITION: Calories: 105 Total Fat: 8g Carbs: 5g Protein: 4g

79..Cauli Mac-n-Cheese

Preparation time: 10 minutes Cooking time: 20 minutes Servings: 4
INGREDIENTS:
- Cauliflower (1 head)
- Butter (3 tablespoons)
- Unsweetened almond milk (.25 cup)
- Heavy cream (.25 cup)
- Cheddar cheese (1 cup)
- Sea salt and freshly cracked black pepper (as desired)

DIRECTIONS:
1. =Slice the cauliflower into small florets and shred the cheese.
2. Prepare the oven to 450º Fahrenheit and cover a baking tray with a sheet of parchment paper or foil.
3. Melt 2 tbsp. of butter in a pan and toss in the florets. Give it a shake of pepper and salt. Place the cauliflower on the baking pan and roast 10 to 15 minutes.
4. Warm up the rest of the butter, heavy cream, milk, and cheese in the microwave or double boiler. Pour the cheese over the cauliflower and serve.

NUTRITION: Calories: 294 Total Fat: 23g Carbs: 7g Protein: 11g

80..Crispy Bacon and Sage Carbonara Zoodles

Preparation time: 10 minutes Cooking time: 30 minutes Servings: 2

INGREDIENTS:
- Butternut squash or pumpkin (1 cup)
- Cauliflower (2 cups)
- Diced organic bacon (1-1.5 cups)
- Zoodles–zucchini noodles (3 cups)
- Turmeric (.25 to .5 teaspoon)
- Salt (as desired)
- Grass-fed butter or ghee (2-3 tablespoons)
- Filtered water/chicken bone broth (.25 cup)
- Fresh sage leaves (1 handful)

DIRECTIONS:
1. Steam the squash/pumpkin and cauliflower in a saucepan until softened.
2. Dice and toss the bacon into a skillet and fry until crispy.
3. When the bacon is ready, remove it from the skillet. Place on a paper-lined dish to drain. Leave the fat in the frying pan.
4. Sauté the sage leaves in the bacon fat until nicely browned and crispy. Transfer the leaves into the plate with the bacon.
5. Toss the zoodles into a saucepan and steam for a few minutes.
6. Combine the cauliflower, cooked squash/pumpkin, turmeric, butter/ghee, salt, and two tablespoons of the broth into a food processor. Pulse until smooth and creamy. Continue adding spoonsful of water/broth to reach the desired sauce consistency.
7. When the zoodles are ready, place them onto two serving platters.
8. Pour the creamy sauce on top, adding a sprinkle of the bacon pieces and crispy sage leaves.
9. Serve and enjoy immediately.

NUTRITION: Calories: 397 Total Fat: 29.5g Carbs: 10.5g Protein: 18.5g

81..Edamame Kelp Noodles

Preparation time: 10 minutes Cooking time: 20 minutes Servings: 2

INGREDIENTS:
- Kelp noodles (1 package)
- Frozen spinach (1 cup)
- Shelled edamame (.5 cup)
- Julienned carrots (.25 cup)
- Sliced mushrooms (.25 cup)
- Sesame oil (1 tablespoon)
- Tamari (2 tablespoons)
- Ground ginger (.5 teaspoon)
- Garlic powder (.5 teaspoon)
- Sriracha (.25 teaspoon)

DIRECTIONS:
1. Soak the noodles in water. Drain well.
2. Use the medium heat temperature setting and toss the sauce fixings in a saucepan. Add the veggies and warm.
3. Stir in the noodles and simmer for two to three minutes. Stir before serving.

NUTRITION: Calories: 139 Total Fat: 9g Carbs: 5g Protein: 8g

82..Chinese Seitan and Celeriac Noodles

Preparation Time: 1 hour 18 minutes Servings: 4

INGREDIENTS:
- 3 tbsp sugar-free maple syrup
- 3 tbsp coconut aminos
- 1 tbsp fresh ginger paste
- ¼ tsp Chinese five spice powder
- Salt and black pepper to taste
- 1 lb seitan, cut into 1-inch cubes
- 2 tbsp butter
- 4 medium large celeriac, peeled and Blade B noodle trimmed
- 1 tbsp sesame oil
- 4 heads baby bok choy, leaves separated
- 2 green onions, chopped for garnishing
- 2 tbsp sesame seeds for garnishing

DIRECTIONS:
1. Preheat the oven to 400 F and line a baking sheet with foil.
2. In a large bowl, mix the maple syrup, coconut aminos, ginger paste, Chinese five-spice powder, salt, and black pepper. Spoon 3 tablespoons of the mixture into a small bowl and reserve for topping. Mix the seitan cubes into the remaining marinade and set aside to marinate for 25 minutes.
3. Meanwhile, melt the butter in a medium skillet and sauté the celeriac until softened, 5 to 7 minutes or until tender. Turn the heat off and set aside.
4. When the marinating is over, remove the seitan from the marinade onto the baking sheet and cook in the oven for 40 minutes or until cooked through.
5. When the seitan is almost ready, heat the sesame oil in a large skillet and sauté the bok choy and zucchini pasta until slightly wilted and tender, 2 to 3 minutes.
6. Transfer to serving bowls and top with the seitan when ready. Garnish with the green onions and sesame seeds.
7. Drizzle the reserved marinade on top and serve warm.

Nutritional Info per Serving: Calories:702, Total Fat:54.9g, Saturated Fat:29.6g, Total Carbs:7g, Dietary Fiber:1g, Sugar:4g, Protein:47g, Sodium:688mg

83..Garlic Pecorino Koodles with Tofu

Preparation Time: 15 minutes Servings: 4

INGREDIENTS:
- 2 tbsp olive oil
- 1 cup sliced tofu
- 4 vegan bacon slices, chopped
- 4 large kohlrabi, peeled and Blade B noodles trimmed
- 6 garlic cloves, minced
- 1 cup cherry tomatoes, halved
- Salt and black pepper to taste
- 7 fresh basil leaves
- 1 cup grated parmesan cheese
- 1 tbsp pine nuts for topping

DIRECTIONS:
1. Heat the olive oil in a large skillet and cook the tofu and vegan bacon until brown, 5 minutes. Transfer to a plate and set aside.
2. Stir in the kohlrabi and cook until tender, 5 to 7 minutes. Mix the garlic into the oil and cook until fragrant, 30 seconds. Then, add the cherry tomatoes, salt, and black pepper; cook for 2 minutes.
3. Mix in the tofu, vegan bacon, basil, and half of the parmesan cheese. Turn the heat off.
4. Dish the food onto serving plates and garnish with the remaining cheese and pine nuts.
5. Serve warm.

Nutritional Info per Serving: Calories:503, Total Fat:50g, Saturated Fat:30.9g, Total Carbs:13g, Dietary Fiber:4g, Sugar:7g, Protein:4g, Sodium:49mg

84..Creamy Tuscan Tofu Linguine

Preparation Time: 35 minutes + overtime chilling time Servings: 4

INGREDIENTS:

For the keto linguine:
- 1 cup shredded mozzarella cheese
- 1 egg yolk

For the creamy Tuscan tofu:
- 2 tbsp olive oil
- 4 tofu
- 1 medium white onion, chopped
- 1 cup sundried tomatoes in oil, drained and chopped
- 1 red bell pepper, deseeded and chopped
- 5 garlic cloves, minced
- 1 tsp dried oregano
- ¾ cup vegetable broth
- 1 ½ cup coconut cream
- ¾ cup grated parmesan cheese
- 1 cup baby kale, chopped
- Salt and black pepper to taste

DIRECTIONS:

For the keto linguine:
1. Pour the cheese into a medium safe-microwave bowl and melt in the microwave for 35 minutes or until melted.
2. Take out the bowl and allow cooling for 1 minute only to warm the cheese but not cool completely. Mix in the egg yolk until well-combined.
3. Lay a parchment paper on a flat surface, pour the cheese mixture on top and cover with another parchment paper. Using a rolling pin, flatten the dough into 1/8-inch thickness.
4. Take off the parchment paper and cut the dough into linguine-like strands. Place in a bowl and refrigerate overnight.
5. When ready to cook, bring 2 cups of water to a boil in medium saucepan and add the keto linguine. Cook for 40 seconds to 1 minute and then drain through a colander. Run cold water over the pasta and set aside to cool.

For the creamy Tuscan tofu:
1. Heat the olive oil in a large skillet, season the tofu with salt, black pepper, and cook in the oil until golden brown on the outside and cooked within, 7 to 8 minutes. Transfer the tofu to a plate and cut into 4 slices each. Set aside.
2. Add the onion, sundried tomatoes, bell pepper to the skillet and sauté until softened, 5 minutes. Mix in the garlic, oregano and cook until fragrant, 1 minute.
3. Deglaze the skillet with the vegetable broth and mix in the coconut cream. Simmer for 2 minutes and stir in the parmesan cheese until melted, 2 minutes.
4. Once the cheese melts, stir in the kale to wilt and adjust the taste with salt and black pepper.
5. Mix in the linguine and tofu until well coated in the sauce.
6. Dish the food and serve warm.

Nutritional Info per Serving: Calories:127, Total Fat:12.7g, Saturated Fat:4.6g, Total Carbs:1g, Dietary Fiber:0g, Sugar:0g, Protein:3g, Sodium:57mg

85..One-Pot Spicy Cheddar Pasta

Preparation Time: 35 minutes Servings: 4
INGREDIENTS:
For the shirataki fettuccine:
- 2 (8 oz) packs shirataki fettuccine

For the spicy cheddar pasta:
- 4 tempeh
- 1 medium yellow onion, minced
- 3 garlic cloves, minced
- 1 tsp Italian seasoning
- ½ tsp garlic powder
- ¼ tsp red chili flakes
- ¼ tsp cayenne pepper
- 1 cup sugar-free marinara sauce
- 1 cup grated mozzarella cheese
- ½ cup grated cheddar cheese
- Salt and black pepper to taste
- 2 tbsp chopped parsley

DIRECTIONS:
For the shirataki fettuccine:
1. Boil 2 cups of water in a medium pot over medium heat.
2. Strain the shirataki pasta through a colander and rinse very well under hot running water.
3. Allow proper draining and pour the shirataki pasta into the boiling water. Cook for 3 minutes and strain again.
4. Place a dry skillet over medium heat and stir-fry the shirataki pasta until visibly dry, and makes a squeaky sound when stirred, 1 to 2 minutes. Take off the heat and set aside.

For the spicy cheddar pasta:
1. Heat the olive oil in a large pot, season the tempeh with salt, black pepper, and cook in the oil until golden brown on both sides and cooked within, 10 minutes. Transfer to a plate, cut into cubes and set aside.
2. Add the onion and garlic to the pan and cook until softened and fragrant, 3 minutes. Season with the Italian seasoning, garlic powder, red chili flakes, and cayenne pepper. Cook for 1 minute.
3. Stir in the marinara sauce, cover the pot and simmer for 5 minutes. Open the lid and adjust the taste with salt and black pepper.
4. Reduce the heat to low and return the tempeh to the sauce as well as the shirataki fettucine, mozzarella cheese and cheddar cheese. Stir until the cheese melts.
5. Dish the food onto serving plates and garnish with the parsley.
6. Serve warm.

Nutritional Info per Serving: Calories:208, Total Fat:20g, Saturated Fat:9.1g, Total Carbs:1g, Dietary Fiber:0g, Sugar:1g, Protein:7g, Sodium:446mg

86..Mushroom Alfredo Zoodles

Preparation Time: 23 minutes Servings: 4

INGREDIENTS:
- 4 tbsp butter
- 4 mushrooms, cut into 1-inch cubes
- Salt and black pepper to taste
- 4 large turnips, peeled and Blade C noodle trimmed
- 3 garlic cloves, minced
- ¾ cup coconut cream
- 1 cup grated parmesan cheese
- 2 tbsp chopped fresh parsley

DIRECTIONS:
1. Melt 2 tablespoons of butter in a large skillet, season the mushroom with salt, black pepper, and cook in the oil until golden brown on both sides and cooked within, 10 minutes. Transfer to a plate and set aside.
2. Melt the remaining butter in the skillet and sauté the turnips until softened, 6 minutes.
3. Add the garlic to the pan and cook until fragrant, 1 minute.
4. Reduce the heat to low and stir in the coconut cream and parmesan cheese until melted. Season with salt, black pepper.
5. Stir in the mushroom and dish the food onto serving plates.
6. Garnish with the parsley and serve warm.

Nutritional Info per Serving: Calories:127, Total Fat:12.7g, Saturated Fat:4.6g, Total Carbs:1g, Dietary Fiber:0g, Sugar:0g, Protein:3g, Sodium:57mg

87..Tomato Kale Eggplant Skillet with Keto Linguine

Preparation Time: 30 minutes + overnight chilling time Servings: 4
INGREDIENTS:
For the keto linguine:
- 1 cup shredded mozzarella cheese
- 1 egg yolk

For the tomato-kale eggplant:
- 3 tbsp olive oil
- 4 large eggplants, cut into 1-inch pieces
- Salt and black pepper to taste
- 1 yellow onion, chopped
- 4 garlic cloves, minced
- 1 cup cherry tomatoes, halved
- ½ cup vegetable broth
- 2 cups baby kale, chopped
- 1 cup grated parmesan cheese for serving
- 2 tbsp pine nuts for topping

DIRECTIONS:
For the keto linguine:
1. Pour the cheese into a medium safe-microwave bowl and melt in the microwave for 35 minutes or until melted.
2. Take out the bowl and allow cooling for 1 minute only to warm the cheese but not cool completely. Mix in the egg yolk until well-combined.
3. Lay a parchment paper on a flat surface, pour the cheese mixture on top and cover with another parchment paper. Using a rolling pin, flatten the dough into 1/8-inch thickness.
4. Take off the parchment paper and cut the dough into linguine strands. Place in a bowl and refrigerate overnight.
5. When ready to cook, bring 2 cups of water to a boil in medium saucepan and add the keto linguine. Cook for 40 seconds to 1 minute and then drain through a colander. Run cold water over the pasta and set aside to cool.

For the tomato-kale eggplant:
1. Heat the olive oil in a medium pot, season the eggplants with salt, black pepper, and sear in the oil until golden brown on the outside. Transfer to a plate and set aside.
2. Add the onion and garlic to the oil and cook until softened and fragrant, 3 minutes.
3. Mix in the tomatoes and vegetable broth, cover and cook over low heat until the tomatoes soften and the liquid reduces by half. Season with salt and black pepper.
4. Return the eggplants to the pot and stir in the kale. Allow wilting for 2 minutes.
5. Divide the keto linguine onto serving plates, top with the kale sauce and then the parmesan cheese.
6. Garnish with the pine nuts and serve warm.

Nutritional Info per Serving: Calories:442, Total Fat:39.9g, Saturated Fat:18.5g, Total Carbs:15g, Dietary Fiber:1g, Sugar:2g, Protein:7g, Sodium:274mg

88..Mustard Tofu Shirataki

Preparation Time: 40 minutes Servings: 4

INGREDIENTS:

For the shirataki angel hair:
- 2 (8 oz) packs angel hair shirataki

For the mustard sauce:
- 1 tbsp olive oil
- 4 tofu, cut into strips
- Salt and black pepper to taste
- 1 medium yellow onion, finely sliced
- 1 medium yellow bell pepper, deseeded and thinly sliced
- 1 garlic clove, minced
- 1 tbsp wholegrain mustard
- 5 tbsp coconut cream
- 1 cup chopped mustard greens
- 1 tbsp chopped parsley

DIRECTIONS:

For the shirataki angel hair:
1. Boil 2 cups of water in a medium pot over medium heat.
2. Strain the shirataki pasta through a colander and rinse very well under hot running water.
3. Allow proper draining and pour the shirataki pasta into the boiling water. Cook for 3 minutes and strain again.
4. Place a dry skillet over medium heat and stir-fry the shirataki pasta until visibly dry, and makes a squeaky sound when stirred, 1 to 2 minutes. Take off the heat and set aside.

For the mustard tofu sauce:
1. Heat the olive oil in a large skillet, season the tofu with salt, black pepper, and cook in the oil until golden brown on the outside and cooked through, 8 to 10 minutes. Transfer to a plate and set aside.
2. Stir in the onion, bell pepper and cook until softened, 5 minutes. Mix in the garlic and cook until fragrant, 30 seconds.
3. Mix in the mustard and coconut cream; simmer for 2 minutes and mix in the tofu and mustard greens. Allow wilting for 2 minutes and adjust the taste with salt and black pepper.
4. Stir in the shirataki pasta, allow warming for 1 minute and dish the food onto serving plates.
5. Garnish with the parsley and serve warm.

Nutritional Info per Serving: Calories:375, Total Fat:32.1g, Saturated Fat:17.8g, Total Carbs:6g, Dietary Fiber:2g, Sugar:4g, Protein:15g, Sodium:237mg

89..Lemon Chicken with Angel Hair Pasta

Preparation time: 5 minutes Cooking time: 20 minutes Servings: 3

INGREDIENTS:
- Shirataki angel hair noodles (2–7-ounce packages)
- Chicken breast (1 pound)
- XCT Oil/another cooking oil (1 tablespoon)
- Organic garlic (1 large clove)
- Dried oregano (.5 teaspoon) or Minced fresh oregano–leaves only (1 teaspoon)
- Himalayan pink salt (.5 teaspoon)
- Large lemon (1)
- Butter or ghee (2 tablespoons)
- Collagelatin/another grass-fed gelatin (1 tablespoon)
- For the Garnish: Fresh oregano–leaves only (1-2 tablespoons)

DIRECTIONS:
1. Zest and juice the lemon into separate containers.
2. Prepare shirataki noodles according to package directions (Rinse for 15 seconds. Boil for 2 minutes in a saucepan of boiling water. Drain the noodles and arrange them in a dry skillet using the medium temperature heat setting. "Dry roast" them for 1 minute). Cool in the pan for 2-3 minutes.
3. In the meantime, warm a large cast-iron skillet using the med-high temperature setting. Pour in the oil.
4. Dice the chicken into small chunks and toss into the skillet with the minced garlic, salt, and dried oregano.
5. Sauté until fully cooked (8-10 minutes). Stir occasionally. Transfer the chicken into a mixing bowl. Set aside.
6. Reduce the skillet temperature setting to medium. Pour in the lemon juice to deglaze the pan. Next, add butter and stir until melted. Whisk in the Collagelatin to finish.
7. Fold the noodles and chicken back into the skillet, tossing to combine.
8. Serve topped with lemon zest and a garnish of fresh oregano.

NUTRITION: Calories: 325 Total Fat: 16g Carbs: 2g Protein: 39g

90..Lemon Garlic Shrimp with Zucchini Pasta

Preparation time: 5 minutes Cooking time: 10 minutes Servings: 4

INGREDIENTS:
- Medium zucchini (4)
- Raw shrimp (1.5 pounds or about 30)
- Olive oil (2 tablespoons)
- Garlic cloves (4)
- Butter or ghee (2 tablespoons)
- Lemon (1 for juice and zest)
- Chicken broth/White wine (.25 cup)
- Chopped parsley (.25 cup)
- Red pepper flakes (a pinch)
- Black pepper and salt (as desired)

DIRECTIONS:
1. Rinse and discard the ends from each zucchini and slice the 'pasta' using a spiralizer. Finely dice the garlic cloves. Peel and devein the shrimp.
2. Warm the olive oil in a skillet using the med-high temperature setting. Toss in the shrimp in a flat layer using a dusting of pepper and salt. Sauté for one minute, but don't stir.
3. Chop and add the garlic and shrimp. Sauté for another one to two minutes on the second side. Transfer the shrimp into a platter.
4. Mix in the butter, lemon juice, zest, white wine, and red pepper flakes into the pan. Simmer for two to three minutes.
5. Sprinkle the parsley and fold in the zucchini pasta. Toss for about 30 seconds to warm it up. Fold in the shrimp and sauté for about one more minute before serving.

NUTRITION: Calories: 306.2 Total Fat: 14.5g Carbs: 8.9g Protein: 27.4g

91..Mushroom Pasta with Shirataki Noodles

Preparation time: 2 minutes Cooking time: 3 minutes Servings: 1

INGREDIENTS:
- Shirataki noodles (2 packages)
- Butter (2 tablespoons)
- Garlic (2 cloves)
- Assorted mushrooms (3 cups)
- Almond flour (1 teaspoon)
- Dried parsley (1 pinch)
- Thick cream (.75 of 1 tub)
- Salt (.25 teaspoon)
- Pepper (.25 teaspoon)
- Olive oil
- For the Garnish: Freshly chopped parsley

DIRECTIONS:
1. Toss the shirataki noodles into a dry frying pan using the medium heat temperature setting. Continue to cook until you hear a whistling sound, indicating the excess moisture leaving the noodles. Transfer to the countertop to cool.
2. Toss the butter into the skillet with the garlic, and sauté for approximately 1 minute or until fragrant.
3. Pour in the oil and add the mushrooms. Sauté for another five minutes, occasionally stirring until the mushrooms are golden in color. Transfer the mushrooms from the pan, leaving the oil behind.
4. Add the almond flour, salt, pepper, dried parsley, and cream. Stir and simmer to combine.
5. Lastly, toss the mushrooms and shirataki noodles into the skillet and combine. Serve right away.

NUTRITION: Calories: 237 Total Fat: 20g Carbs: 4g Protein: 6g

92..Pesto Shirataki Noodles–Vegan

Preparation time: 2 minutes Cooking time: 3 minutes Servings: 1
INGREDIENTS:
- Shirataki noodles (2–8-ounce packages)
- Fresh basil (2 cups packed)
- Minced garlic (1 clove)
- Pine nuts (.25 cup)
- Nutritional yeast (.25 cup)
- Salt (1 pinch)
- Olive or pistachio oil (.25 cup)

DIRECTIONS:
1. Drain and rinse the shirataki noodles thoroughly. Boil for two to three minutes or microwave for one minute.
2. Combine the remainder of the fixings in a food processor, drizzling in olive oil while the motor is running.
3. Mix the pesto with the prepared noodles and serve.

NUTRITION: Calories: 190 Total Fat: 19g Carbs: 1g Protein: 2g

93..Salmon Pasta

Preparation time: 5 minutes Cooking time: 5 minutes Servings: 2
INGREDIENTS:
- Coconut oil (2 tablespoons)
- Smoked salmon (8 ounces)
- Zucchini (2)
- Keto-friendly mayo (.25 cup)

DIRECTIONS:
1. Melt the oil in a skillet using the med-high temperature setting.
2. Add the salmon and sauté for 2-3 minutes or until lightly browned.
3. Prepare the zucchini using a peeler or spiralizer to make the noodle-like strands. Toss into the skillet and sauté for 1-2 minutes.
4. Mix in the mayo before serving.

NUTRITION: Calories: 470 Total Fat: 42g Carbs: 3g Protein: 21g

94. Salmon and Avocado Pesto Zucchini Noodles

Preparation time: 5 minutes Cooking time: 5 minutes Servings: 1
INGREDIENTS:
- Skinless wild salmon (4-ounce)
- Black pepper and salt
- Pesto (1 tablespoon)
- Large zucchini (1)
- Avocado (.25 of 1)
- Cherry tomatoes (3)

DIRECTIONS:
1. Warm the oven in advance to 425º Fahrenheit.
2. Prepare a baking tray with a layer of parchment baking paper.
3. Trim the noodles in a processor using the D blade. Slice the avocado and slice the tomatoes into halves.
4. Place the salmon on the paper and sprinkle using the pepper and salt.
5. Bake until the salmon flakes and are opaque (8-10 min.).
6. In the meantime, toss the pesto with the zucchini noodles until they're covered.
7. Arrange the noodles in a pasta dish and garnish using avocados, tomatoes, and salmon before serving.

NUTRITION: Calories: 320 Total Fat: 20g Carbs: 10g Protein: 29g

95. Stuffed Shells Florentine

Preparation time: 15 minutes Cooking time: 10 minutes Servings: 8

INGREDIENTS:
- 1 package (12 ounces) jumbo pasta shells
- 1 egg, lightly beaten
- 2 cartons (15 ounces each) ricotta cheese
- 1 package (10 ounces) frozen chopped spinach, thawed and squeezed dry
- 1/2 cup grated Parmesan cheese
- 1/2 teaspoon salt
- 1/2 teaspoon dried oregano
- 3 breadsticks, optional

DIRECTIONS:
1. Cook pasta shells according to package directions. Meanwhile, in a large bowl, combine the egg, ricotta cheese, spinach, Parmesan cheese, salt, oregano and pepper. Drain shells and rinse in cold water; stuff with spinach mixture.
2. Place shells in a greased 13-in. x 9-in. baking dish. Pour spaghetti sauce over shells. Cover and bake at 350 degrees for 30-40 minutes or until heated through. Serve with breadsticks if desired.

NUTRITION: Calories: 292 Total Fat: 10g Carbs: 38g Protein: 15g

96. Stuffed Shells with Arrabbiata Sauce

Preparation time: 30 minutes Cooking time: 20 minutes Servings: 12

INGREDIENTS:
- 1 package (12 ounces) jumbo pasta shells
- 1 pound ground beef or turkey
- 1/2 pound fresh chorizo or bulk spicy pork sausage
- 1/2 large onion, chopped (about 1 cup)
- 3 garlic cloves, minced
- 1 package (10 ounces) frozen chopped spinach, thawed and squeezed dry
- 3/4 teaspoon salt, divided
- 1/2 teaspoon pepper, divided
- 1 carton (15 ounces) part-skim ricotta cheese
- 3/4 cup grated Parmesan cheese
- 2 large eggs, lightly beaten
- 1/4 cup chopped fresh basil
- 2 tablespoons chopped fresh parsley

Arrabbiata sauce:
- 2 tablespoons olive oil
- 6 ounces sliced pancetta, coarsely chopped
- 2 teaspoons crushed red pepper flakes
- 2 garlic cloves, minced
- 2 jars (24 ounces each) marinara sauce
- 1-1/2 cups shredded part-skim mozzarella cheese

DIRECTIONS:
1. Preheat oven to 400 degrees. Cook pasta according to package directions for al dente. Drain and rinse in cold water.
2. In a large skillet, cook and crumble beef and chorizo with onion and garlic over medium heat until meat is no longer pink and vegetables are tender, 6-8 minutes; drain. Stir in spinach, 1/2 teaspoon salt and 1/4 teaspoon pepper. Transfer to a bowl; cool.
3. Stir ricotta and Parmesan cheeses, eggs, basil, parsley and remaining salt and pepper into meat mixture. For sauce, in a saucepan, heat oil over medium heat. Add pancetta; cook and stir until golden brown, 6-8 minutes. Add pepper flakes and garlic; cook and stir 1 minute. Add marinara sauce; bring to a simmer.
4. Spread 1 cup sauce into a greased 13x9-in. baking dish. Fill pasta shells with meat mixture; place in baking dish, overlapping ends slightly. Top with remaining sauce. Sprinkle with mozzarella cheese. Bake until heated through and cheese is melted, 20-25 minutes.

NUTRITION: Calories: 198 Total Fat: 14g Carbs: 24g Protein: 14g

97. Sunday Shrimp Pasta Bake

Preparation time: 30 minutes Cooking time: 25 minutes Servings: 8

INGREDIENTS:
- Three (3) cloves of mincedgarlic
- Two (2) tablespoons of butter
- Two (2) medium zucchini
- A quarter teaspoon salt to taste
- A quarter teaspoon pepper
- A quarter cup of parmesan cheese

DIRECTIONS:
1. 12 ounces uncooked vermicelli
2. 1 medium green pepper, chopped
3. 5 green onions, chopped
4. 6 tablespoons butter, cubed
5. 6 garlic cloves, minced
6. 2 tablespoons all-purpose flour
7. 2 pounds cooked medium shrimp, peeled and deveined
8. 1 teaspoon celery salt
9. 1/8 teaspoon pepper
10. 1 pound process cheese (Velveeta), cubed
11. 1 can (10 ounces) diced tomatoes and green chilies, drained
12. 1 can (4 ounces) mushroom stems and pieces, drained
13. 1 tablespoon grated Parmesan cheese

NUTRITION: Calories: 558 Total Fat: 25g Carbs: 42g Protein: 42g

98. Creamy Zoodles

Preparation time: 20 minutes Cooking time: 25 minutes Servings: 8

INGREDIENTS:
- 8 ounces uncooked spiral pasta
- 8 ounces Johnsonville TM ; Fully Cooked Smoked Sausage Rope, cut into 1/4 inch slices
- 2 medium sweet potatoes, peeled and cut into 1/2 inch cubes
- 1 cup chopped green pepper
- 1/2 cup chopped onion
- 2 tablespoons olive oil
- 1 teaspoon minced garlic
- 1 can (14-1/2 ounces) diced tomatoes, undrained
- 1 cup heavy whipping cream
- 1/4 teaspoon salt
- 1/4 teaspoon pepper
- 1 cup shredded cheddar cheese

DIRECTIONS:
1. Cook pasta according to package directions. Meanwhile, in a large skillet, cook the sausage, sweet potatoes, green pepper and onion in oil over medium heat for 5 minutes or until vegetables are tender. Add garlic; cook 1 minute longer. Drain.
2. Add the tomatoes, cream, salt and pepper. Bring to a boil; remove from the heat. Drain pasta; stir into sausage mixture. Transfer to a greased 13x9-in. baking dish. Sprinkle with cheese.
3. Bake, uncovered, at 350 degrees for 25-30 minutes or until bubbly. Let stand for 5 minutes before serving.

NUTRITION: Calories: 198 Total Fat: 6g Carbs: 4g Protein: 4g

99. Swiss Cheese Lasagna

Preparation time: 60 minutes Cooking time: 40 minutes Servings: 12

INGREDIENTS:
- 1 pound ground beef
- 1 large onion, chopped
- 1 garlic clove, minced
- 3 cups water
- 1 can (12 ounces) tomato paste
- 2 teaspoons salt
- 1/2 to 1 teaspoon dried rosemary, crushed
- 1/4 teaspoon pepper
- 1 package (8 ounces) lasagna noodles
- 8 ounces sliced Swiss cheese
- 1-1/2 cups (12 ounces each) 4% cottage cheese
- 1/2 cup shredded part-skim mozzarella cheese

DIRECTIONS:
1. In a large skillet, cook the beef, onion and garlic over medium heat until meat is no longer pink; drain. Stir in the water, tomato paste, salt, rosemary and pepper. Bring to a boil. Reduce heat; simmer, uncovered, for 30 minutes.
2. Meanwhile, cook lasagna noodles according to package directions; drain. In a greased 13-in. x 9-in. baking dish, layer a third of the meat sauce, noodles and Swiss cheese. Repeat layers. Top with cottage cheese and the remaining Swiss cheese, noodles and sauce. Sprinkle with mozzarella cheese.
3. Cover and bake at 350 degrees for 30 minutes. Uncover; bake 10-15 minutes longer or until bubbly. Let stand for 10 minutes before serving.

NUTRITION: Calories: 275 Total Fat: 11g Carbs: 23g Protein: 20g

100. Swiss Macaroni

Preparation time: 20 minutes Cooking time: 30 minutes Servings: 6

INGREDIENTS:
- 1 package (7 ounces) elbow macaroni
- 1 jar (2 ounces) diced pimientos, drained
- 2 large eggs, lightly beaten
- 1 cup half-and-half cream
- 1 small onion, chopped
- 2 tablespoons minced fresh parsley
- 1-1/2 teaspoons salt
- 1/8 teaspoon pepper
- 1 cup soft bread crumbs
- 1 cup shredded Swiss cheese
- 1/4 cup butter, melted

DIRECTIONS:
1. Cook macaroni according to package directions; drain and place in a greased 11x7-in. baking dish. Stir in the pimientos. In a large bowl, combine the eggs, cream, onion, parsley, salt and pepper.
2. Pour over macaroni mixture. Sprinkle with bread crumbs and cheese; drizzle with butter. Bake, uncovered, at 350 degrees for 30 minutes or until golden brown.

NUTRITION: Calories: 269 Total Fat: 14g Carbs: 24g Protein: 10g

101. Tangy Meatballs Over Noodles

Preparation time: 25 minutes Cooking time: 50 minutes Servings: 8

INGREDIENTS:
- 1 egg, lightly beaten
- 1/3 cup milk
- 1/4 cup seasoned bread crumbs
- 1 tablespoon dried minced onion
- 1 teaspoon salt
- 1-1/2 pounds ground beef
- 2 cans (14-3/4 ounces each) beef gravy
- 1/2 cup packed brown sugar
- 1/4 cup cider vinegar
- 3/4 teaspoon ground ginger
- 1/4 teaspoon ground cloves
- 1 package (12 ounces) egg noodles

DIRECTIONS:
1. In a large bowl, combine the first five ingredients. Crumble beef over mixture and mix well. Shape into 1-1/2-in. balls. Place meatballs on a greased rack in a shallow pan. Bake, uncovered, at 350 degrees for 20 minutes; drain.
2. With a slotted spoon, transfer meatballs into a greased 2-1/2-qt. baking dish. Combine gravy, brown sugar, vinegar, ginger and cloves; pour over meatballs. Cover and bake 30 minutes longer or until meat is no longer pink. Meanwhile, cook noodles according to package directions; drain. Serve with meatballs.

NUTRITION: Calories: 435 Total Fat: 14g Carbs: 51g Protein: 26g

102. Tasty Chicken Noodle Casserole

Preparation time: 20 minutes Cooking time: 35 minutes Servings: 8
INGREDIENTS:
- 1 package (16 ounces) egg noodles
- 1 medium sweet red pepper, chopped
- 1 large onion, chopped
- 1 celery rib, chopped
- 1/4 cup butter, cubed
- 2 garlic cloves, minced
- 1-1/2 cups sliced fresh mushrooms
- 3 tablespoons all-purpose flour
- 3 cups chicken broth
- 3 cups half-and-half cream
- 2 packages (8 ounces each) cream cheese, cubed
- 12 cups cubed cooked chicken
- 1 to 1-1/2 teaspoons salt

Topping:
- 1 cup finely crushed cornflakes
- 2 tablespoons butter, melted
- 1 tablespoon canola oil
- 3 tablespoons minced fresh parsley
- 1/2 teaspoon paprika

DIRECTIONS:
1. Cook noodles according to package directions; drain. In a large skillet, sauté the red pepper, onion and celery in butter until tender. Add garlic; cook 1 minute longer. Add mushrooms; cook 2-3 minutes or until tender. Remove vegetables with a slotted spoon; set aside.
2. Add flour to the skillet; stir until blended. Gradually add broth. Bring to a boil; cook and stir for 2 minutes or until thickened. Reduce heat. Gradually stir in cream. Add the cream cheese; cook and stir until cheese is melted. Remove from the heat.
3. In a large bowl, combine the chicken, salt, noodles, vegetables and cheese sauce. Transfer to two ungreased shallow 3-qt. baking dishes.
4. Combine topping ingredients. Sprinkle over top. Cover and bake at 350 degrees for 20 minutes. Uncover; bake 15-20 minutes longer or until bubbly.

NUTRITION: Calories: 399 Total Fat: 19g Carbs: 24g Protein: 31g

103. Tempting Turkey Casserole

Preparation time: 15 minutes Cooking time: 25 minutes Servings: 3

INGREDIENTS:
- 3 ounces uncooked spaghetti, broken into 2-inch pieces
- 1/2 cup process cheese sauce, warmed
- 1/4 cup 2% milk
- 1-1/2 cups frozen chopped broccoli, thawed
- 3/4 cup cubed cooked turkey
- 1/3 cup canned mushroom stems and pieces, drained
- 1 tablespoon pimientos, chopped
- 1/8 to 1/4 teaspoon onion powder
- 1/8 teaspoon poultry seasoning

DIRECTIONS:
1. Cook spaghetti according to package directions. Meanwhile, in a small bowl, whisk cheese sauce and milk. Add the broccoli, turkey, mushrooms, pimientos, onion powder and poultry seasoning. Drain pasta; add to broccoli mixture.
2. Transfer to a 1-qt. baking dish coated with cooking spray. Cover and bake at 350 degrees for 25-30 minutes or until heated through.

NUTRITION: Calories: 313 Total Fat: 12g Carbs: 29g Protein: 22g

www.ingramcontent.com/pod-product-compliance
Lightning Source LLC
Chambersburg PA
CBHW081118080526
44587CB00021B/3646